Population Change and Health Care

Population Change and Health Care

Study of Karnataka

C.M. Lakshmana

RAWAT PUBLICATIONS
Jaipur | New Delhi | Bangalore | Hyderabad | Guwahati

ISBN 978-81-316-0432-8

The publication of this book was financially supported by ICSSR and the responsibility for the facts stated, opinions expressed, or conclusions reached, are entirely that of the author. ICSSR accepts no responsibility for them.

ICSSR Consultant: A.M. Khan, Professor and Head of Social Science, National Institute of Health & Family Welfare (NIHFW), New Delhi.

Published by
Prem Rawat for **Rawat Publications**
Satyam Apts., Sector 3, Jawahar Nagar, Jaipur 302 004 (India)
Phone: 0141 265 1748 / 7006 Fax: 0141 265 1748
E-mail: info@rawatbooks.com
Website: www.rawatbooks.com

New Delhi Office
4858/24, Ansari Road, Daryaganj, New Delhi 110 002
Phone: 011 2326 3290

Also at *Bangalore, Hyderabad* and *Guwahati*

Typeset by *d'lines* DTP SERVICES, Jaipur
Printed at Nice Printing Press, New Delhi

Dedicated to

Late Prof. V.K.R.V. Rao

a great philosopher

and

Founder, Institute for Social & Economic Change (ISEC), Bangalore

Contents

Foreword

Karnataka has made remarkable progress in social and economic spheres during the twentieth century. The industrial development of the state is now widely acclaimed and the city of Bengaluru is recognized, nationally and internationally, as a major centre of information technology. On the other hand, the major demographic changes that have occurred in the state have received relatively less attention in popular media. This is surprising given that the pioneering Mysore Population Study covered a major portion of the state and this was followed later by a number of major research efforts, including the Bangalore Population Study, the Karnataka Fertility Survey, and the three rounds of the National Family Health Survey in the state. It is now abundantly clear that Karnataka has moved from a regime of high fertility and high mortality at the beginning of the twentieth century, to one of moderately low mortality and nearly replacement level low fertility by the end of it, thereby completing the demographic transition. In the process, as it happens inevitably, population grew, initially slowly, then rapidly, especially during the second half of the century, and now the growth rate has begun to decline. The population will continue to grow, on account of population momentum, for some time, but at a very low rate and the population trajectory is expected to turn downwards by the middle of the present century. The major demographic changes in the state, especially in fertility, occurred during the last two-three decades of the twentieth century. The impact is seen on the age structure, with the share of the working ages rising notably. Consequently, Karnataka now has the opportunity to derive the demographic dividend.

Karnataka is known for wide diversity. This is seen in its physiographic and agro-climatic conditions as well as social settings. Besides, initially, the administrative structures also varied as the state was formed by combining Kannada-speaking areas of a number of provinces and states. Naturally, economic development has not been uniform across various regions of the state and regional imbalances have been a major concern for successive state governments. Similarly, demographic changes have also varied spatially within the state. Child mortality has fallen to very low levels in some regions, particularly in the coastal districts, while some others show moderately high levels. The same applies to fertility, varying from below replacement level to moderately high. Though changes have occurred and are continuing to occur in all the regions of the state, some have been lagging thereby creating notable differentials. This is most probably a passing phase, as those lagging would eventually catch up with the leaders but there are implications in terms of growth differentials.

Given the diversity in the state, it is desirable to see how the demographic picture varies across the state. How are the various regions placed in terms of population growth and structure? Are there pockets of low growth? Does the age structure differ spatially? What is the tempo of urbanization? Addressing these questions is important to observers of the social and economic scene and to policy makers and planners in the state.

Dr. Lakshmana has tried to answer some of these questions in his present book. While analyses of spatial variations in India generally examine inter-district differences, this work goes a step deeper and looks at data at the taluk level. Many districts of Karnataka have vast areas and population well over two million and are thus larger than many countries in the world. One does then expect substantial differences in conditions within the districts and the present analysis brings this out quite clearly. The approach adopted in this work is indeed rewarding.

While mortality has gradually fallen over time, especially after the first quarter of the twentieth century, the level is still well over that of the developed world. There is thus need to strengthen efforts to improve the health conditions in the state. This calls for a detailed examination of health conditions and, in particular, health care infrastructure in the state. This book has addressed this issue. Moreover, special attention has been paid to the health needs of children,

In India, the scheduled tribes are a marginalized section on account of the relative isolation in which they live and thereby suffer from lack of access to various opportunities and even basic services. Dr. Lakshmana has rightly devoted space to the study of this large section of the society.

The present work contributes to an understanding of spatial variations in the state of Karnataka by looking at the dimensions of population growth and health care. It is expected that researchers studying other dimensions of Karnataka's society and economy would find this line of research useful and contribute to a comprehensive and deep understanding of social, economic, and demographic aspects of Karnataka's development.

Prof. P.M. Kulkarni

Jawaharlal Nehru University, New Delhi

Preface and Acknowledgements

In India, the last decade of the 20th century, known for the onset of the LPG era in the country, witnessed not only the extensive economic development but also the expansion of infrastructural facilities in the country. As a result, there have been lots of changes in the entire process of population movements, especially in the growth and distribution. In view of this, the studies of population have acquired immense value in understanding different dimensions of a given area/region. Its impact on population growth and distribution has also drawn the attention of researchers to study the different characteristics of population. The global population has been increasing rapidly since the past two decades and is currently adding about 77 million people a year. Similarly, the population of India has also been rising at a rapid pace. However, due to initiatives taken by the Department of Health and Family Welfare, Government of India and the states through various policies and programmes, the population growth rate showed a declining trend in the decade 1991–2001. As of 2001, India with only 2.4 per cent of the global surface area sustains a population of 102.8 crore, accounting for about 16.7 per cent of the world population. If the current trends of population increase continue, India will become the most populous country in the world and push back China by 2045.

In Karnataka, the socio-economic development as well as the growth and distribution of population vary from district to district and one region to another. The growth of population in Karnataka as elsewhere in India is a fundamental obstacle and the chief determinant factor in the process of economic development. There have been several studies on population over the years both at national and international levels. However, most of these studies focused mainly on the general population growth and distribution. The present work is an attempt at better understanding of the micro analysis with regard to population change in Karnataka.

I am grateful to the Institute for Social and Economic Change (ISEC), Bangalore for providing me an opportunity to work and make use of this academic platform to improve my knowledge in the study of population. Firstly, I dedicate this work to late Prof. V.K.R.V. Rao, founder director of ISEC. I am personally indebted to Prof. R.S. Deshpande, the present director of the Institute for his whole-hearted support. I would also like to place on record my gratefulness to Prof. Gopal Kadekodi and Prof. N. Jayaram, the then directors, ISEC.

My heartfelt thanks are also due to Dr B. Eswarappa, Professor of Geography, my teacher and research guide, without whose able guidance, this work would not have been possible. I owe a debt of gratitude to my family, especially my wife Nandini, and children Darashan and Vandana, for their moral support.

The publication of this book has been possible due to financial support provided by the ICSSR, New Delhi. In particular, I am grateful to Dr. Prem Prakash Pandey, Deputy

Director, ICSSR, for the same. My thanks are also due to Prof. K.S. James, Head, PRC, and the entire academic and non-academic staff of Population Research Centre, and other colleagues at ISEC.

Finally, I am grateful to Rawat Publications, Jaipur, for the publication of the book in a nice manner within the stipulated time frame.

C.M. Lakshmana

1

The Geographic, Social and Economic Profile of Karnataka

Availability of natural resources, favourable environmental and infrastructural facilities in a given region, have played a pivotal role in the general distribution of population. Rich natural resources of Karnataka like black cotton soils in the north, generation of power and growth of industries and agricultural development in the Southern Maidan region have influenced to a great extent the growth and distribution of population. The hilly terrain of the Western Ghats has also influenced the natural growth and distribution of population. The coastal region with its narrow strip of fertile land witnessed industrial development due to the availability of hydropower from west flowing rivers. This in conjunction with the quality of population of the region made for its unique characteristics. The phenomenal growth of information technology and other knowledge-based industries particularly in and around Bangalore (Bengaluru) metropolis, have had its impact on the growth and distribution of population, in the region.

Birth rate, death rate and migration are the three important determinants of population growth and change. The global population increased from 3.85 billion in 1971 to 6.1 billion in 2000 and is currently (2006) growing by 77 million people a year. Most of the growth is concentrated in developing regions, with nearly two-thirds in Asia and Pacific. In India, population has grown steadily from 1901, except for a decrease in the decade 1911–1921. The total population of India was 23.8 crore in 1901 which increased to 36.1 crore in 1951 and 102.7 crore in 2001. India has got only 2.4 per cent of the total land area in the world but, it is the home for 16.7 per cent of the world's population.

The population of Karnataka increased from 19 million (1901) to 52.7 million (2001) during the century. Further, it is estimated to increase to 60.4 million by the year 2011. However, the growth rate in the decade 1991–2001 has slightly decreased, i.e., from 21.12 per cent in 1991 to 17 per cent in 2001. This can be attributed to the economic development and family welfare programmes initiated by both central and state governments in the previous decades.

It is evident from the Five-Year Plan documents that provision for expenditure on family planning in the total plan outlay was quite lower in First Five-Year Plan at 0.03 per cent and 3.1 per cent in the Ninth Plan (1997–2002). The progress achieved in sterilization and Intra-Uterine Device (IUD) for birth control programmes in India indicates that, the cumulative number of sterilizations and IUD insertions increased from 8,08,27,473 in 1991 to 12,49,86,025 in 2001 and from 4,64,37,174 in 1991 to 10,71,37,641 in 2001. Similar progress can be seen in sterilizations and IUD insertions. There was an absolute increase of cumulative sterilizations from 1,89,000 in 1981–82 to 62,23,600 in 2001 and IUD insertions from 55,000 in 1981–82 to 46,23,700 in 2001.

Over the years, a large number of studies have emerged in Karnataka, offering explanation for the growth of population by districts, most of them being made either by census department or independent researchers, but there have been no attempts to study population issues at the 'taluk' level in Karnataka. Research studies on population growth including its various demographic dimensions are plenty at the international scenario (Wilbur Zelinsky, 1966; Colin Clark, 1970;

Simon Kuznets, 1974; Robert Goodland, 1992 and Ann Florini, 2003). Even in the Indian context particularly for states like Haryana, Punjab, Rajasthan etc., there have been some attempts (Mehta, 1970; Srinivasan, 1981; Patil, 1978; Singh, Premi, Bhatia and Bose 1989; Jhingan et al., 2003).

The work on *Population Growth in Kerala* (1965) edited by Kapur and George, gives the overall demographic characteristics of the population of Kerala. This work addresses many important issues like social, economic and medical implications of the past growth of population of Kerala. Further it embodies an insightful discussion on relevant demographic issues pertaining to Kerala.

The work *Population, Family and Culture* edited by Patil (1978) deals with some qualitative aspects of population research in the country. The qualitative dimensions of population research are critically examined in the study by various experts in the field.

The study *Agricultural Change and Growth of Rural Population in Karnataka* by Bhattacharjee (1978) briefly explains the trends in population growth at the district level in Karnataka. During the decade 1951–61 population growth was faster in rural areas as compared to the decade 1961–71. The relatively lower growth witnessed during the decade 1961–71, was due to faster rate of growth of urban population in the state, associated with rural-urban migration.

Population Structure of Indian Cities (Singh, 1985) has gone into the details of factors influencing the changes in population. This investigation with focus on urban population in Bihar dwells on different aspects of population during inter-censual decades in the cities of Bihar.

The work *Population Trends in the Brahmaputra Valley* (1985) by Goswami, provides information on population for the use of demographers, policy makers, population experts, planners and economic historians interested in perusing scientific study of the behavioural dynamics of population in the Brahmaputra Valley.

In his work the author identifies the major factors responsible for the growth and variations in the population of Assam for the period 1881–1931. The study attempts to supply the gaps in the population statistics of Assam, particularly in the field of fertility, mortality and migration rates.

A recent study on "Fertility Transition in Karnataka" (2004, ISEC) by Sekher and Raju, gives an in-depth analysis of population growth across districts.

The book *Regional Population Growth: A Case Study of Rajasthan* (Mehta, 1970) throws light on the population growth rates in different regions of Rajasthan. The study has shown that, dry regions have been consistently showing high rate of population growth; it is opposed to plain and hilly regions which have registered a slower pace of population growth. Also growth has been found distributed more evenly in hilly and plain regions than in dry region.

Over the years, child population trends have helped project potential needs for education, childcare, health care and other services for children. Most of the studies on child population have drawn attention towards either adverse sex-ratios or gender discrimination (Sekher, 2006). However, researchers and demographers have focused on the general population growth and distribution and no attention has been given to understand the child population under age 0–6, in India as well as Karnataka. Therefore, there is no relevant literature available on child population under age 0–6 both at national and state levels.

However, at the international level a study was carried out in 2001 by William to trace the status of children in the United States. In this study the author has tried to trace the relative change in the growth rate of child population over the past two decades. An effort has been made in this study to trace the demographic shift in 1990s by studying the growth in the number of children between the years 1990 and 2000. Children in the USA accounted for 40 per cent of the total population in 1900, but only 26 per cent in 2000. This is the result of two demographic trends. First, the movement towards smaller families over the century intended fewer children being born late in the century as compared to earlier century. Second, increase in life expectancy led to a larger adult population in 2001.

Studies at the micro level, play a crucial role in understanding ground realities as also formulating plans for development. The investigation aims to bring out a detailed picture of the dimensions of population in a given set of regions in order to highlight the overall scenario of population growth across taluks in Karnataka, and bring out the major changes in the growth rate.

Population as a renewable resource plays a crucial role in any developmental initiative in a given region. In the present situation, the state of Karnataka needs long-term policies and programmes both for development and correction of inter-district variations in socio-economic development. The study on population change across taluks in Karnataka is expected to be helpful in taking initiatives for the reduction of population growth for achieving further development in socio-economic spheres in Karnataka.

The present study has certain limitations. First, investigation excludes four taluks in Bangalore Urban and seven taluks in Bangalore Rural districts, as these two districts had witnessed highly polarized urban growth and consequent unusual concentration of population with unique demographic characteristics as compared to other parts of the state. Hence, the investigation has been limited to 164 out of 175 taluks in Karnataka. Second, the data on birth rate, death rate and migration are not available at taluk level. Therefore, some related variables have been selected which directly or indirectly affect population growth. These include, female literacy, ethnic group of population (social variables), percentage of urban population and irrigated area (economic variables) registered births, child-woman ratio and population covered under family welfare programmes like contraceptives and IUD insertions (demographic variables). A study also explains the changing child population under age 6 years in Karnataka in the last two decades. Further it is evident from census data that the growth of STs in Karnataka was highest (44.70%) in the country in the decade of 1991–2001. Hence, the study also focuses in understanding the growth and its trends of ST population in India by states.

The Geographic and Population Profile

Geographically, Karnataka has been divided into three natural regions as Eastern (where it is subdivided into Northern and Southern Maidan), Malnad and Coastal regions. However, for the study purpose the districts of Karnataka have been divided into four regions (see Figure 1.1). For administrative purpose it is further divided into four divisions, viz., Bangalore, Belgaum, Gulbarga and Mysore and consists of a total of 175 taluks. There are inter-regional and inter-district differences in social and economic development, which have also influenced the emergence in different patterns of population growth across the state. For example, dry regions have consistently shown higher rates of population growth, whereas plains and hilly regions have recorded relatively lower growth. Given this background, the study lays special emphasis on the need to consider talukwise growth and distribution of population in Karnataka during the decades 1981–1991 and 1991–2001. Further, the study has gone into the details of both negative and positive growth as also the social, economic and demographic causes behind such changes.

Figure 1.1
Location Map of Karnataka – 2010

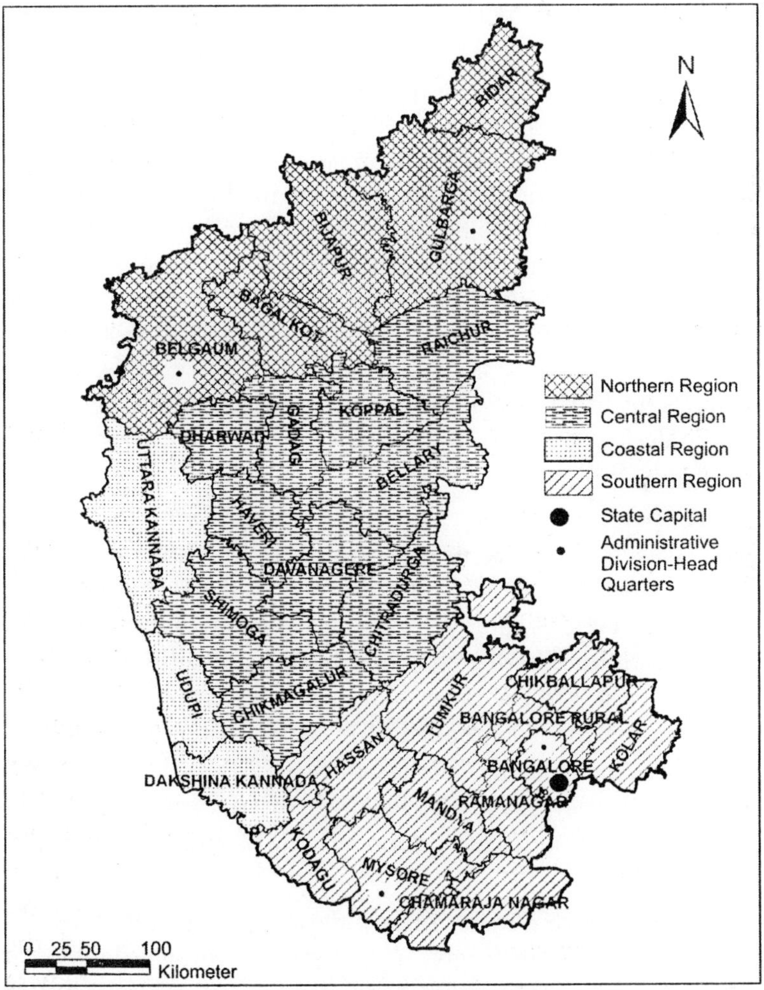

The state of Karnataka lies to the south-western part of peninsular India. The latitudinal extend between 11°31′ and 18°45′N, and longitudinal extend between 74°12′N and 78°40′ E. It has an area of 1,91,791 sq km (5.83%) and 5,27,33,598 (5.13%) of population in India (2001). The state is fairly endowed with good land resources. It has 54.65 per cent of net sown area in the total geographical area, and 25.39 per cent of net area irrigated to the net area sown (2001).

Geographically, the southern part has undulating central hill ranges with red soils. Northern Karnataka is a relatively plain region with black cotton soil. The western part of Karnataka is having fairly good forests in Western Ghats; has plantation agriculture and hydroelectric projects on rivers like Sharavathi, Kali etc. As per 2001 census the state has 67 per cent of literacy and a per capita income of Rs 17,847 at current prices. The demographic indicators of the state, like birth rate, death rate and sex-ratio are 25, 8 and 964 respectively. The birth rate is below the all-India level, i.e., 26.1. The male-female ratio in the state is well above the national average at 933.

As per 2001 census, the total urban population of the state was 34 per cent and similarly the average urban population per district in southern region has highest with 4.54 per cent (Table 1.1). The lowest average urban population per district was reported in coastal districts, i.e., 2.45 per cent. On the other hand, the highest district average rural population was reported in northern region with 5.28 per cent. And coastal districts have relatively lower average rural population (2.9%). The average district rural population in central and southern region was 3.02 and 2.95 per cent respectively.

The average density of population of the state was 275 per sq km. Interestingly, the district average density in southern region was absolutely double (574 persons per sq km) as compared to the state average density of 275. And more or less the district average density of population in the coastal region was same as compared to the state average. The northern and central region districts had lower density with 241 and 236 per sq km, respectively.

Table 1.1

Geographic and Population Profile of Karnataka by Region and Districts (2000–2001)

	Districts	*%age of geographical area to the total*	*%age of urban population to the total*	*%age of rural population to the total*	*Density of population 2001*	*Population growth rate 1991–2001*
Northern Region	Bidar	2.84	1.92	3.32	276	20
	Belgaum	6.99	5.64	9.18	314	17
	Gulbarga	8.46	4.75	6.53	193	21
	Bijapur	5.47	2.21	4.04	172	18
	Bagalokot	3.43	2.66	3.36	251	19
	Total	27.19	17.17	26.43	241	19
Coastal Region	Uttar Kannada	5.37	2.16	2.77	132	11
	Dakshin Kannada	2.38	4.06	3.35	416	14
	Udupi	2.02	1.15	2.6	286	7
	Total	9.77	7.37	8.71	278	10.66

Cont'd...

Cont'd...

Central Region	Chitradurga	4.40	1.53	3.56	179	15
	Davanagere	3.09	3.02	3.58	302	15
	Raichur	3.56	2.34	3.58	241	22
	Koppal	3.75	1.1	2.86	166	25
	Chickmagalur	3.76	1.24	2.63	158	12
	Dharwad	2.22	4.91	2.07	376	17
	Gadag	2.43	1.91	1.8	209	13
	Haveri	2.51	1.66	3.27	298	13
	Shimoga	4.42	3.18	3.07	193	13
	Bellary	4.41	3.94	3.78	240	22
	Total	34.55	24.83	30.21	236	16.7
Southern Region	Bangalore	1.14	32.07	2.23	2979	35
	Hassan	3.55	1.07	1.89	253	10
	Kodagu	2.14	0.42	1.36	133	12
	Bangalore Rural	1.18	1.07	1.89	323	12

Cont'd...

Cont'd...

Mandya	2.59	1.57	4.24	355	7
Mysore	3.57	5.47	4.75	383	15
Chikkaballapur	2.22	1.23	2.66	0	0
Kolar	2.07	2.25	2.82	307	14
Tumkur	5.53	2.82	5.95	243	12
Ramanagar	1.85	1.2	2.34	0	0
Chamarajnagar	2.66	0.82	2.34	189	9
Total	28.5	50	32.47	574	14
Karnataka	**100**	**34**	**66**	**275**	**17.25**

Source: Government of Karnataka, 2007, Karnataka Socio-Economic Indicators, 2005, Department of Economics and Statistics, Bangalore.

The total growth rate of population in Karnataka in the decade 1991–2001 was 17.25 per cent. However, apart from the northern region the average growth of population in rest of the region was lower than the state average of 17.25 per cent. There was slightly higher rate of population growth reported in the northern region (19%).

According to 2001 census, the total birth rate of Karnataka was 19.47 per 1,000 population. The average birth rate in the region of coastal and central region was higher than the state average of 19.47. A similar picture can be seen in Table 1.2, with regard to death rates. The state average death rate was 6.99 per 1,000 population. Whereas, central and coastal regions have death rates of 7.53 and 7.91 respectively which is above the state average. But the southern (6.35) and northern (6.64) regions have reported lower death rates than the state average of 6.99. If we come to the status of sex-ratio, i.e., total females per 1,000 males, the coastal region has shown highest sex-ratios with 1,040 females per 1,000 males, which is highest among four natural regions in Karnataka. Interestingly, except northern region, the rest of the two regions had higher sex-ratios than the state average of 964 females per 1,000 males. The sex-ratios of the southern and northern regions were 968 and 965 respectively.

The total literacy of Karnataka in the year 2001 was 67 per cent. The lowest rate of literacy has been reported in northern region with 57.88 per cent. However, one can observe that the coastal region has achieved higher literacy, which is above the state average (67%) with 80.4 per cent. The literacy rate of the coastal region was 80.4 per cent. The southern and central regions had a literacy rate of 66.23 and 64.54 per cent respectively. Generally, Karnataka has achieved higher male literacy with 75.29 per cent. Further it was also higher in the general as well as in female literacy in the year 2001.

Out of four regions in the state, the coastal region has higher male literacy at 80.4 per cent. Relatively, the northern region has lower male literacy of 70.16 per cent. The central and southern regions had male literacy rate of 75.02 and 75.29 per cent respectively. Similarly, the total female literacy in Karnataka was 56.9 per cent. Of this, the coastal region reported higher female literacy of 73.63 per cent which is above the state average. But it was below the state average in the case of northern (45.22%) and central region (53.53%). It is observed from Table 1.2 that the female literacy was slightly higher (57.4%) than the state average of 56.9 per cent in the northern region.

Table 1.2

Demographic, Social and Economic Profile of Karnataka by Region and District (2001)

Demographic Profile

	Districts	*Birth rate*	*Death rate*	*Sex-ratios*	*Literacy rate*	
					Total	*Male*
Northern Region	Bidar	17.5	5.15	948	60.9	72.5
	Belgaum	20.79	6.9	959	64.2	75.7
	Gulbarga	15.09	5.62	964	50	61.8
	Bijapur	20.95	7.03	948	57	69.9
	Bagalokot	21.83	8.53	977	57.3	70.9
	Total	19.23	6.64	959	57.88	70.16
Coastal Region	Uttar Kannada	21.53	7.45	970	76.6	84.5
	Dakshin Kannada	21.51	7.32	1023	83.4	89.7
	Udupi	22	8.98	1127	81.2	86.2
	Total	21.68	7.91	1040	80.4	86.8
Central Region	Chitradurga	21.79	7.5	955	64.5	74.7
	Davanagere	19.72	7.16	951	67.4	76.4
	Raichur	19.43	8	980	48.8	61.5
	Koppal	22.68	6.94	982	54.1	68.4
	Chickmagalur	19.67	7.04	984	72.2	80.3
	Dharwad	24.35	8.47	948	71.6	80.8

Cont'd...

Cont'd...

	Gadag	19.78	8.22	968	66.1	79.3
	Haveri	24.22	6.81	942	68.8	77.6
	Shimoga	19.9	7.8	977	74.5	82
	Bellary	21.09	7.38	969	57.4	69.2
	Total	21.26	7.53	965	64.54	75.02
Southern Region	Bangalore	16.59	6.47	906	83	87.9
	Hassan	18.23	6.37	1005	68.6	78.4
	Kodagu	21.16	4.45	996	78	83.7
	Bangalore Rural	16.19	5.44	953	69.7	79.1
	Mandya	16.79	7.34	985	61	70.5
	Mysore	18.06	6.43	965	63.5	70.9
	Chikkaballapur	0	0	0	62.8	73.2
	Kolar	16.63	5.78	970	62.8	73.2
	Tumkur	20.22	7.32	966	67	76.8
	Ramanagar	0	0	0	61.3	75.5
	Chamarajnagar	18.2	7.55	968	50.9	59
	Total	18	6.35	968	66.23	75.29
	Karnataka	**19.47**	**6.99**	**964**	**67**	**76.1**

Social and Economic Profile

	Districts	*Female*	*%age of SC population to the total*	*%age of ST population to the total*	*District income (in lakh rupees at current prices) (2005–06)*	*Per capita income (In Rs at current prices) (2005–06)*
Northern Region	Bidar	48.8	19.89	12.13	212660	13361
	Belgaum	52.3	10.96	5.78	886681	19858
	Gulbarga	37.9	22.92	4.92	584602	17624
	Bijapur	43.5	18.5	1.66	294648	15392
	Bagalokot	43.6	15.17	4.85	343464	19625
	Total	45.22	17.4	5.86	464411	17172

Cont'd...

Cont'd...

Coastal Region	Uttar Kannada	68.5	7.53	1.76	300185	20932
	Dakshin Kannada	77.2	6.91	3.32	762852	37943
	Udupi	75.2	6.09	3.74	312931	26558
	Total	73.63	6.84	2.94	458656	28477
Central Region	Chitradurga	53.8	22.17	17.54	285089	17728
	Davanagere	58	18.61	11.71	386590	20374
	Raichur	35.9	19	18.15	289811	16382
	Koppal	39.6	15.48	11.59	281996	22253
	Chickmagalur	64	20.43	3.6	339143	28059
	Dharwad	61.9	8.23	4.39	449123	26424
	Gadag	52.5	14.14	5.6	199831	19409
	Haveri	57.4	12.19	8.84	262188	17197
	Shimoga	66.9	16.41	3.41	376335	21627
	Bellary	45.3	18.46	17.99	745535	34715
	Total	53.53	16.51	10.28	3615641	22416
Southern Region	Bangalore	77.5	13.02	1.32	4105403	59277
	Hassan	59	18.11	1.54	327361	17947
	Kodagu	72.3	12.29	8.41	220832	37996
	Bangalore Rural	59.8	21.92	5.13	541929	27188
	Mandya	51.5	14.02	0.97	307553	16460
	Mysore	55.8	17.71	10.27	682242	24383
	Chikkaballapur	52.2	23.91	11.97	0	—
	Kolar	52.2	28.61	4.91	456546	16992
	Tumkur	56.9	18.34	7.5	466541	17038
	Ramanagar	51.7	18.54	17.35	0	—
	Chamarajnagar	42.5	24.61	10.99	144405	14117
	Total	57.4	19.18	7.3	725281	23139
	Karnataka	**56.9**	**16.2**	**6.55**	**14566476**	**26015**

Source: Government of Karnataka, 2007, Karnataka Socio-Economic Indicators, 2005, Department of Economics and Statistics, Bangalore.

As per 2001 census, Karnataka has about 16 per cent of SCs and almost 7 per cent of STs in its total population. Taking into account its proportion in the total population, the average SC population was highest in the southern and central region with 19.18 per cent and 16.51 per cent respectively. However, the coastal region has relatively lower proportion with 6.84 per cent as compared to the other part of Karnataka. Similarly, the total proportion of ST population in the total population of Karnataka was 7 per cent. This was seen as higher in the central (10.28%) and southern (7.3%) regions in Karnataka. The highest proportion of ST population in the total population is observed in district of Bellary (18%) and lowest proportion was reported in the district of Mandya (0.97%).

The total per capita income of the state in the year 2005–06 at current prices was Rs 26,015, in which the average total income at regional level was relatively lower than the state average in the northern region (Rs 17,172). On the other hand, the coastal region has higher per capita income with Rs 28,477 which is higher than the state average. The southern and central regions have a per capita income of Rs 23,139 and Rs 22,416 respectively (Table 1.2). Similarly, if we come to the districtwise income of Karnataka in the year 2005–06, the total net income of the state was Rs 1,45,66,476. For the various reasons the average district income by regions was reported to vary from one region to another as well as from one district to another. The central region which consists of Bellary, which is mainly involved in mining, in the recent decades has shown higher average district income with Rs 36,15,641. The average district income in the southern region was Rs 7,25,281 lakh and this is followed by northern region (Rs 4,64,411 lakh) and Rs 4,58,656 lakh in the central region.

2

Theories of Population

Before going into the main theme of the book, let us understand some theories of population in brief. I have summarized here some of the important theories of population propounded by eminent scholars like Malthus, Edwin Cannan, Thomas Doubleday, Dumont's, Marx and Leibenstein. We can classify these theories into four as: (i) the Malthusian and neo-Malthusian theory, (ii) the optimum theory of population, (iii) the biological theories of population, (iv) the social and economic theories of population, and (v) the theory of demographic transition. Let us begin with the Malthusian theory of population.

Thomas Robert Malthus published his famous book *Essay on the Principle of Population* (as it affects the future improvement of society) in 1798. In his theory the main objective was about food supply and population increase. His observation was that the pressure of increasing population on the food supply would destroy perfection and there would be misery in the world. His theory of population was based on the three postulates: (i) food is essential for man's existence, (ii) the passion between the sexes is essential and it will nearly remain in its present state, and (iii) the law of diminishing returns operates in agriculture.

The Malthusian doctrine is stated as follows: (a) There is a natural sex instinct in human beings to increase at a fast rate. As a result, population increases in geometrical progression and, if unchecked, doubles itself every 25 years. (b) On the other hand, the food supply increases in a slow arithmetical progression due to the operation of the law of diminishing returns based on the supposition that the supply of land is constant. (c) Hence, he further states that as population increases in geometrical progression and the food supply in arithmetical progression, population tends to outrun food supply.

In Malthusian words, "It is the constant tendency in all animated life to increase beyond the nourishment prepared for it." Thus, an imbalance is created which leads to overpopulation. However, the doctrine was widely discussed and criticized during the 19th and early 20th century. Some of them are:

(i) Mathematical form of the theory was wrong.

(ii) Failed to foresee the opening up of new areas in relation to increased production of food.

(iii) Applied a static economic law to a period of time. About his third postulation, the law of diminishing returns operating in agriculture was criticized on the ground that Malthus could not foresee unprecedented increase in scientific knowledge and agricultural inventions over a period of time. Consequently, the food supply has increased much faster than arithmetical progression. He has been proved wrong not only in the advanced countries but also in the developing countries like India with the 'green revolution' in 1960s.

(iv) Neglected the manpower aspect in population.

This has been criticized by Cannan in the following words: "A baby comes to the world not only with a mouth and a stomach, but also with a pair of hands."

This implies that an increase in population means an increase in manpower which may tend to increase not only agricultural but also industrial production and thus makes the country rich in terms of equitable distribution of wealth and income.

(v) Population not related to food supply to total wealth.

(vi) Importance given to only food grains for livelihood.

(vii) Increase in population being the result of declining death rate.

(viii) Empirical evidence proves the theory wrong.

(ix) Preventive checks do not pertain to moral restraint.

(x) There is a difference between sexual desire and desire for children.

(xi) Sexual desire is not the same in human beings; it differs from person to person and depends on age, health and physical and environmental factors.

(xii) Positive checks are not due to overpopulation.

(xiii) Malthus is a false prophet.

(xiv) Not relevant to modern population problems.

The main difference between the Malthusian and neo-Malthusian doctrines was that Malthus favoured celibacy and self-restraint in controlling the population growth. Whereas the neo-Malthusians favoured artificial means of birth control. The neo-Malthusians also did not accept the Malthusian vice that the sexual urge is the same in all human beings. They believed that it differs from person to person, depending on the age, health, psychology and environment as has been already mentioned. In this view, one can conclude that the views of neo-Malthusians on birth control have been accepted by all countries. But a number of developed countries like France, fear a secular decline in their population. The use of contraceptives has led to moral degradation of society.

The optimum theory of population was propounded by Edwin Cannan in his book *Wealth* published in 1924 and it was popularized by Robbins, Dalton and Carr Saunders. This theory was based on seven assumptions: (i) the natural resources of a country are given at a point of time but they change over time, (ii) there is no change in techniques of production, (iii) the stock of capital remains constant, (iv) the habits and tastes of the people do not change, (v) the ratio of working population to total population remains constant even with the growth of population, (vi) working hours of labour do not change, and (vii) modes of business organization are constant. According to these assumptions, the theory of optimum population is that ideal size of population which provides the maximum income per head. Any rise or diminution in the size of population above or below the optimum level will diminish income per head. Given the stock of natural resources, the technique of production and the stock of capital in a country, there is a definite size of population. It corresponds to the highest per capita income. Other things being equal, any deviation from this optimum population, will lead to a reduction in the per capita income.

The optimum theory of population is superior to the Malthusian theory on the following justification:

(i) The Malthusian law is a general study of the population problem as it is applicable to all countries irrespective of their economic conditions.

(ii) The Malthusian theory is a static concept which applies to a period of time. The optimum theory is a dynamic one, because over a period of time the per capita income may rise with the expansion in output due to improvements in knowledge, skill, capital, equipment and other elements in production.

(iii) The Malthusian doctrine is simply theoretical in nature and is devoid of all practical considerations.

(iv) The Malthusian theory of population is based on the unrealistic assumption of the niggardliness of nature.

(v) The optimum theory of population does not suffer from any pessimism; rather it adopts an optimistic and realistic attitude towards the problem of population when it relates population to the wealth of the country.

Biological Theories of Population

Thomas Doubleday, a social philosopher, and also an economist, expresses his views regarding various natural laws which govern population. According to him, the rate of population increase will be less when the quantity of food supply is greater. According to Doubleday, fertility is affected by leanness in all plants and animals. An overfed plant can be reviewed only when the plants are exhausted either by ringing the bark or by extreme lopping or the trenching of the roots. Besides, the sterility in plant life is possible when the application of fertilizers is excessive. Further, he believes that thin birds or animals give birth to more issues, while bulky or fat birds or animals give birth to fewer ones. Similarly, this becomes true about trees and plants. It means that fertility depends on the fatness of living beings, according to Doubleday. Further, he observes that high fertility has been found in those persons who are vegetarians, or who eat more rice or whose staple diet is rich, whereas fertility will be low in non-vegetarian persons.

He classifies the society into three groups: (i) The first group includes those who are in a state of affluence and are well supplied with luxuries. Their number always increase. (ii) The second group consists of the poor people who have less supply of food. Their number is increasing rapidly. (iii) The third group comprises those people who are between two opposite states and who fall under the average income group with good food or a normal diet and do not overwork and yet are not idle. Their number is stationary. Doubleday further explains that, "the rich produce less children as the fertility is found to be less amongst them, and therefore, their wealth will be distributed among a few people".

Josue De Castro expressed his views in his famous book *The Geography of Hunger* regarding the correlation between fertility and the consumption of protein. Castro accepted the findings of R.J. Solankar who conducted experiments on rats in 1920. In these experiments Solankar found that with the increase in protein consumption in diet, the fecundity would decrease and vice versa with low protein content. His experiment led to the following conclusions:

(i) when 10 per cent protein was given to a female rat, per mated female rat gave 23.3 births;

(ii) when 18 per cent protein was given to each female rat, per mated female rat gave 17.4 births; and

(iii) when the quantity of protein was increased to a level of 22 per cent to each female rat, the birth per mated female rat got reduced to 13.8 births. From these experiments Castro came to the conclusion that fatness was affected by the consumption of protein. Fatness increases with the protein rich diet, leading to lower fertility. This concept of Castro is similar to the Doubleday's diet theory that the rate of population increase is influenced by food supply.

According to Castro, balanced food is not available to the poor, and therefore, they always get less protein from food which results in sluggish liver function. Consequently, the estrogens in women's body cannot be neutralized, and with the increase in estrogens, the reproductive capacity of a woman increases. As a result it led to high birth rate. Therefore, as compared to the rich, the birth rate among the poor people (due to chronic hunger, malnutrition) is high. But in the case of acute hunger, sexual activity goes down.

Castro reflects on the issues with reference to India, in that, out of the total number of children born in India, almost 50 per cent suffer from starvation and die before they reach the age of marriage. On the basis of data collected for different countries, relating to the association of fertility with consumption many experience chronic hunger, i.e., malnutrition, disease or early death. According to him, the fertility rates can be reduced only if more attention is paid to the production of food crops than commercial crops which are made available to the poor people. He pointed out that to eradicate chronic hunger, priority should be given to the problem of balanced food. Efforts should be made to bring more lands under the plough with improved farming methods and extensive cultivation.

Michael Thomas Sadler's Destiny Theory

Thomas was an economist and a British social reformer. He was a contemporary of Malthus. According to him, the law which regulates the growth of animals and plants is primarily the same as the law which regulates the growth of human population. In his opinion, the fecundity of human beings is in the inverse ratio of the condensation of their number. Moreover, the fertility rate decreases with an increase in the density of population. He states that in the agriculture based or pastoral countries, where the density of population is low, the fertility rate of the population is high. In such countries, people have the capacity to work hard, and hard working people give birth to more children. With the passing of time, when there is industrialization, and the population becomes more civilized and literate, the density of population increases. Here people tend to limit the size of family and in such social economic conditions, they feel happier with prosperity.

Sadler was a great critic of Malthus and did not accept his view that population would increase in geometrical progression and food supply in arithmetical progression. According to him, such increase of population and food supply in mathematical terms just cannot happen, because when population increases, density too will increase. Further, he says that when density increases, the capacity to produce more children goes down, and thus with the increase in density the fertility rate declines. He argues that population adjusts itself with the times.

He did not accept the Malthus view that positive checks by nature would take place with the growth of population. Being optimistic he tried to establish a link between population and food supply. He was of the view that if the fertility rate of population increased, people would be able to produce more food (supply) and that the population would get adjusted to it. He further argued that when the density of population increased the unhealthy atmosphere would also increase. As a result, it influenced the increase in the death rates. When the death rate is high, it leads to increase in the birth rate; this happens to compensate for the loss of population.

Herbert Spencer's Biological Theory

Herbert Spencer was a famous English philosopher and sociologist; he propounded the biological theory of population in his book *The Principles of Biology*. Spencer argues that fecundity deceases when the complexity of life increases. According to him, changes in the growth of population occur due to natural change in the reproductive capacity of human beings. Therefore, his theory has been known as a natural theory of population and is similar to the theory of Sadler and Doubleday. Spencer believed that "there exists antagonism between individuation and genesis". At working pace when an individual does work hard for his personal development, the desire for reproduction deceases. In other words, when more energy has been utilized for one's self-development, the energy available for reproduction will be less and consequently the population growth will be less.

He has classified four different situations which explain the relation between individuation and genesis: (i) the individuation will automatically be low when there is high genesis as in the poor, (ii) the genesis will be low when there is high individuation as in the rich, (iii) the individuation will improve when the genesis is low, and (iv) the genesis will be high when the individuation is low. We find less individuation and more genesis among poor people.

Spencer's theory of population is based on the theory of evolution. According to Spencer, the fertility rate is higher in small creatures. In the words of Spencer "The minutest organisms multiply asexually (without sex) in their millions". Many small cells do not reach the maturity period. If this happens and small cells grow twice or thrice in number, population will rapidly increase and multiply itself. Small compound cells increase in thousands, while big compound cells in hundreds and still bigger cells lose their productive capacity. In the same manner, Spencer explains the fertility of human beings. According to him, people can be divided into three groups as: (i) poor people who live a simple life whose fertility is high, (ii) middle class people whose fertility is correspondingly low, and (iii) people who live a developed or complex life whose fertility is fairly low.

According to him, in societies where people, especially women, are educated and belong to rich families, their reproductive power is low, as compared to the poor who are uneducated and whose reproductive power is high. Spencer believed that if population increases we get more manpower through which natural resources can be exploited and the socio-economic and cultural standards of the people raised.

Thus, in his opinion, increase in population is beneficial rather than harmful. Also he believed that the determining factor for birth and death rate is longevity. The expectancy of life increases and the death rate decreases when there is improvement in the quality of life; it becomes more complex and further reduces the death rates. He, therefore, suggested increases in life expectancy in order to reduce the birth rate.

Pearl and Reed's Longistic Curve

This theory was suggested by Quetlet in 1835. He argued that the growth of population tended to slow down with the increase in density of population. But, people did not give recognition to it. However, the credit goes to Raymond Pearl and Lowwell Reed in popularizing this Longistic curve theory of population growth. Pearl's study was based on two experiments: in the first experiment, he gave gelatinized banana pudding (in constant quantity) to the fruit flies in a bottle. In the beginning, the fertility rate rapidly increased. But with the increased number of fruit flies the density in the bottle increased and with the increase in density, the fertility rate of fruit flies decreased and subsequently it became negligible. In the same manner, Pearl also found through the second experiment, that with the increase of hens in their pens, density went up; hens produced fewer eggs as the space became less. Thus, fertility rate came down with more density.

On the basis of these experiments, he concluded that the fertility rate of human population would come down whenever the density went up. Based on this experience he further states that there will be a high birth rate among poor people or in labour colonies.

Corrado Ginnis's Biological Theory

Corrado Ginnis, a sociologist was born in Italy in 1884. He had deep interest in the study of population changes which has affected the evolution of society and that of a nation. In his opinion, population increases due to high fertility and as a result, social and economic problems become complex. Along with that, industrial and trade problems also become more complex and as such the pressure of population is ultimately reduced through war or colonization or both. According to him, first the fertility rate declines among the rich, after that when the energetic and prolific poor people enter the rich class, their fertility also decreases when the whole society or country becomes rich, and consequently there will be a decline in population growth due to the weakening of the reproductive instinct. Ginnis concludes that it is a providential mechanism to eliminate those family stocks which have fulfilled the cycle of their evolution.

Social and Economic Theories of Population

There have been several social and economic theories of population by sociologist and economist thinkers. However, I have discussed here only three important theories as explained by the great scholars: Dumont, Marx and Leibenstein.

Dumont's Theory of Social Capillarity

Theory of social attraction or aversion to a thing is known as social capillarity. According to Dumont, there are three principles of population that are related to the stages of social development, they are: (i) in the preventive stage the Malthusian theory of population applies where human beings live like animals; (ii) in the intermediate stage, Quillard's principle of population applies, according to this "population proportions itself automatically". In such a society, population increases as food supply increases because population can produce food itself, hence, positive checks do not become necessary; and (iii) in a modern civilized society,

Dumont applies his social capillarity principle. In such a society, every individual wants to achieve higher economic and social status. For this, a small family is imperative, because one cannot climb high on the social ladder with the burden of more children on its back. When an individual earns more income and wealth, his ambition for better position and higher social prestige goes up, and consequently, the number of children decreases. Thus, social capillarity has direct relation with social development, and further, birth rate and social capillarity are inversely related to each other. Dumont claims that socialism leads to the destruction of social capillarity.

Karl Marx's Theory of Surplus Population

Karl Marx, the famous author of *Das Kapital*, did not submit any specific theory of population like Malthus. He disregards totally the Malthusian views that population increases in geometric progression and food supply in arithmetical progression. His views about population growth are based on his theory of surplus value.

Capitalism, according to Marx, is divided into two classes: the workers who sell their 'labour power', and the capitalist who wins the 'means of production' (industrial unit). Labour power is like any other commodity. The labourer sells his labour for its value; and its value, like the value of any other commodity, is the amount of labour required to produce labour power. This is determined by the number of necessary hours, for its production. But the value of commodities, necessary for the subsistence of the labourer, is never equal to the value of the produce that labourers produce. If a labour works for ten hours a day, but it takes him six hours labour to produce goods for covering his subsistence, he will be paid wages equal to six hours. The difference worth of four hours of labour goes into the capitalist pocket in the form of profit. Marx calls this unpaid work 'surplus value'.

According to Marx, this surplus value leads to capital accumulation. The capitalist's main aim is to increase the surplus value in order to increase his profit. He further explains how productivity and labour are related. In the market if the productivity of labour increases, the labourer produces the same commodity in less time. This raises the surplus value and the capitalists profit. The increase in the productivity of labour requires a technological change that helps in increasing total output besides lowering the cost of production. He introduces labour saving machines which in turn increase labour productivity. This process of replacing labour by machines creates an industrial reserve army which keeps increasing as capitalism develops. The industrial reserve army is the surplus labour. The larger will be the industrial reserve army, the larger the surplus population and worse are the conditions of the employed labourers. This is because the capitalists can dismiss dissatisfied and troublesome workers and replace them with the ranks of the reserve army. Capitalists are also able to cut down on wages to a semi-starvation level and raise more surplus value resulting in more surplus population.

Leibenstein's Motivational Theory of Population Growth

Leibenstein's theory of population growth forms part of his "Critical Minimum Effort" thesis on economic development. It is based on the empirical evidence that the rate of population growth is a function of the level of per capita income which, in turn, depends on the level of economic development. Leibenstein's view is similar to Dumont's "Social-capillarity Thesis" which states that with the increase in per capita income, the desire to have more children as productive agents declines. This means that as per capita income rises with economic development, the fertility rate declines. Similarly, the mortality rate also declines, as there is improvement in public health care measures with economic development. But, the decline in the mortality rate is fast as compared, to the decline in the fertility rate. This creates a 'fertility gap' which continues to widen for quite some time.

This theory concludes that at the low level of per capita income, there is a greater motivational force on the part of parents to have an additional child as a productive agent and a source of security. This motivation continues up to a particular level of per capita income. But, as per capita income increases beyond a particular level, the motive to have an additional child declines because the direct and indirect costs of bringing up an extra child increase while productive and security utilities decline. These sequences are closely related to the different stages of economic development.

Theory of Demographic Transition

The theory of 'demographic transition' was propounded by W.S. Thomson and F.W. Notestein, and this has been explained in three stages. But, here, I have given due weightage in presenting the further version of the five stages of population growth as explained by C.P. Blacker. The theory of demographic transition explains the effects of changes in birth and death rates on the growth rate of population. According to E.G. Dolan, "Demographic transition refers to population cycle that begins with a fall in the death rate, continues with a phase of rapid population growth and concludes with a decline in the birth rate".

This theory states that every country passes through different stages of population development. This has been explained by C.P. Blacker in terms of different stages, viz., (i) the high stationary phase marked by high fertility and mortality rates, (ii) the early expanding phase marked by high fertility but dealing mortality, (iii) the late expanding phase with declining fertility but mortality dealing more rapidly,

(iv) the low stationary phase with low fertility balanced by equally low mortality, and (v) the dealing phase with low mortality, lower fertility and an excess of deaths over births. According to Blacker, this stage continued in West Europe approximately up to 1840 and in India and China till 1990.

In the first stage, the country is backward and is characterized by high birth and death rates with the result that the growth rate of population is low. Here, people mostly live in rural areas and their main occupation is agriculture which is in a state of backwardness. The tertiary sector consisting of transport, commerce, banking and insurance is underdeveloped. All these economic and social factors are responsible for a high birth rate in the country. In the second stage of demographic transition, the economy enters as the phase of economic growth. The agriculture and industrial sector productivity increases and means of transport develop. There is greater mobility of labour and education expands. People get more and better quality food products. Medical and health care facilities are expanded; as a result, modern drugs are used by the people. All these factors bring down the death rate. But the birth rate is almost stable. According to Blacker, 40 per cent of the world population was in this stage up to 1930; and many countries in Africa are still in this stage.

The birth rate starts declining accompanied by death rates dealing rapidly. With better medical facilities the survival rate of children increases. People are not willing to support large families and use contraceptives to limit their family size. This is the scenario of third stage of demographic transition. According to Blacker, 20 per cent of the world population was in this stage in 1930. In the fourth stage, the fertility rate declines and trends to equal the death rate so that the growth rate of population is stationary. The level of people's living conditions rises with increasing income. Education expands and inspires the entire society. People discard old customs, dogmas and beliefs. Men and women prefer to marry late. People are ready to adopt family planning devices to limit their family size. All these factors tend to reduce the birth rate, further, which along with an already low death rate, brings the dealing growth rate of population. The advanced countries of the world are passing through this stage of population growth.

In the last stage of demographic transition death rates exceed birth rates and the population growth declines. A continuing decline in birth rate, when it is not possible to lower the death rate, further in the advanced countries, leads to a 'declining' stage of population. France appears to be approaching this stage.

By conclusion, the theory of demographic transition is the most acceptable theory of population growth. It does not lay emphasis on food supply like the Malthusian theory nor does it develop a pessimistic outlook towards population growth. It is also superior to the optimum theory of population. The biological theories study the problem of population growth simply from the biological angle. In view of all this the demographic transition theory is superior to all the theories of population because it is based on the actual population growth trends in the developed countries of Europe.

3

An Overview of Population Growth Transition in Karnataka

Characteristics of population growth and its distribution across regions in Karnataka are unique, and largely determined by the socio-cultural and economic features specific to the regions as well as the districts. As already discussed in the previous chapter, distinct geographies of the different regions in Karnataka have had its decisive impact on the socio-economic development of the respective region. For example, black soil in the northern districts of Dharwad, Bijapur, Bellary, Belgaum, Raichur, Gulbarga and Chithrdurga has had its impact on the developmental activities of this region. Similarly, forest-based activities common to Western Ghats have determined the development pattern of the western region districts of the state. On the other hand, irrigation, hydroelectric and even navigation potential of Tungabadra, Cauvery, Pennar and Palar rivers which led to establishment of diverse industries, have immensely contributed to the development of southern districts of Karnataka. The airport and seaport at Mangalore in Dakshin Kannada has been a strong catalyst for the economic development of the state, particularly the coastal region.

Population Size and Growth in Karnataka

As per 1901 census (pre-independence period) the total population of Karnataka was 13.54 million; it increased to 19.40 million by 1951 (post-independence period). Further the total population of Karnataka increased to 37.13 million by 1981, reached 52.73 million by 2001, and is expected to reach 61.52 million by the year 2011 (see Table 3.1). In regard to the growth rate of population in Karnataka, as can be seen from Figure 3.1, it has been increasing sharply throughout the period under review except for the decade of 1911–1921. This is mainly attributed to epidemics like cholera, malaria and plague which devastated this region in that decade and caused both degradation of public health and reduction of population size and growth. Figure 3.1 shows that the growth rate of population was significantly low at 3.6 per cent in the decade 1901–1911, but witnessed a steady increase in the following decades, i.e., 1921–1931 (9.38%) to 1971–1981 (26.74%).

Figure 3.1

Decadal Growth of Population in Karnataka

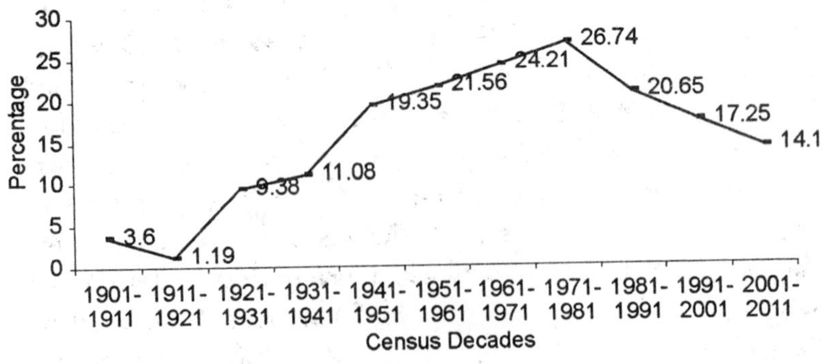

However, as a result of the health and family welfare programmes initiated as part of the national strategy for controlling population growth, the state witnessed a major demographic shift in the last quarter of 20th century. This downward shift is reflected in the population growth figures for the decade 1981–1991; the growth rate came down from 26.74 per cent in the decade 1981–1991 to 20.65 per cent in decade 1991–2001. Table 2 contains more details of this demographic shift and its impact on the population growth in Karnataka.

Table 3.1

Selected Demographic Indicators of Karnataka

Year	*Total population (in million)*	*Growth rate of population (in%)*	*Birth rate*	*Death rate*	*Fertility rate*	*Infant mortality rate*
1961	23.58	21.57	21.2	8.1	—	61.6
1971	29.30	24.26	33	12.4	—	95
1981	37.13	26.75	27.6	9.2	3.7	69
1991	44.97	21.12	26.9	8.5	3.1	77
2001	52.73	17.25	22.2	8.4	2.2	58
2011	61.52	14.10	—	—	—	—

Source: Socio-economic Indicators, Directorate of Economic and Statistics, Government of Karnataka, Bangalore.

Birth rate for the year 1961 was 21.2 per 1000 population; it increased to 27.6 in 1981, but came down to 22.2 in 2001. But if we look at death rates for Karnataka, unlike birth rate, it has remained stable in the past decades. In the subsequent years, fertility rates also came down, i.e., from 3.7 in 1981 to 2.2 in 2001. The growth rate of population in Karnataka also varied across the religious groups. For example, the growth rate of Hindu population in Karnataka for the year 1961 was 15.32 per cent, whereas the growth rate of other religious groups was higher. This can be seen from Table 3.2. There are several reasons for the higher growth rate of population among non-Hindu religious groups in

Karnataka as well as at the national level. However, this chapter focuses on the various demographic, social and economic aspects that influenced the growth of population in Karnataka. This is discussed in detail in the next chapters.

Table 3.2

Decadal Growth of Religion Population (1991–2001)

Religion	*Hindu*	*Muslim*	*Christian*	*Sikh*	*Buddhist*	*Jains*
Population Growth (in %)	15.32	23.48	17.41	51.72	438.67	26.53

Source: Statistical Abstract, India 2004–05.

Rural-Urban Share in Total Population

Historically Karnataka economy was predominantly agriculture-based, and a significant share of population was rural, and Karnataka's contribution to the national economy was quite significant. But, over the years other activities like industrialization, urbanization and infrastructural development got primacy altering the shape of economic development in the state, particularly since the 1980s. As a result, the state currently has a higher share of urban dwellers in the total population. As can be seen from Figure 3.2, in 1961 about 77.7 per cent of the population was rural. Since then, rural population has declined steadily. The proportion of rural population in 2001 was 66 per cent, which is expected to decrease to 65 per cent by 2011. However, thanks to the rapid strides in agricultural development in the recent decades, despite the burgeoning urbanization, proportion of rural population in the total population has stabilized during the recent decades. This is particularly attributable to the strong agricultural base created by introduction of modern agricultural technology, expansion of irrigation, land-reclamation, establishment of agro-based industries, etc. The decline in the proportion of rural population seems to have been slowed down significantly; the share of urban population is expected to be about 65 per cent by 2011. However, there has been a continuous increase in the proportion of urban population in the total (see Figure 3.2).

Figure 3.2

Proportion of Rural Population in the Total Population of Karnataka

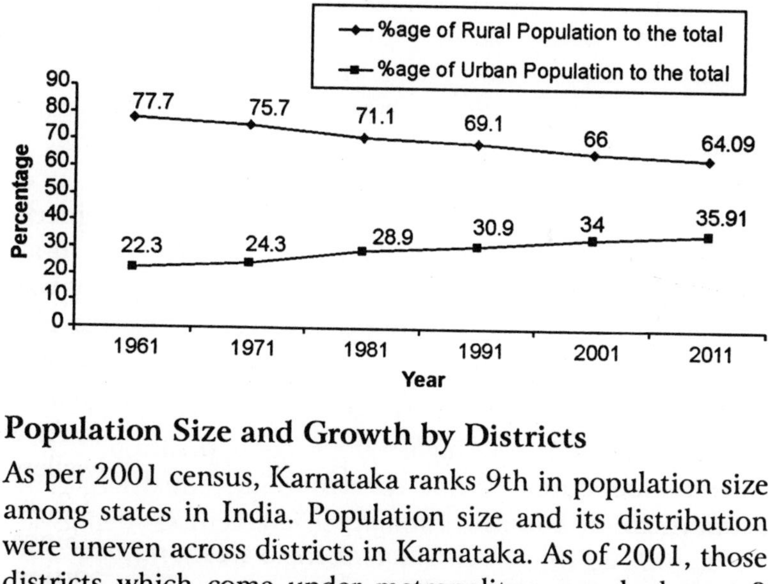

Population Size and Growth by Districts

As per 2001 census, Karnataka ranks 9th in population size among states in India. Population size and its distribution were uneven across districts in Karnataka. As of 2001, those districts which come under metropolitan area had over 3 million population each, and districts which are categorized as second tier cities, i.e., Bellary, Tumkur, Kolar and Mysore (categorized as second tier cities) had 2 to 3 million of population each. In the recent decades, the share of urban population in these districts has become higher than rural population. Employment opportunities created in the wake of globalization and industrialization in both public and private sector have been attracting more and more people to urban areas. This influx to urban areas is not without consequence: the number of unemployed youth in urban agglomerations has been rising alarmingly. Most of the rural youths are naturally absorbed in the urban unorganized/informal sector. As a result, in Karnataka, even second tier cities/ districts are fast emerging as centres of business and entrepreneurial activity. This is particularly true of the southern districts of the state. As is evident from the recent experience of Karnataka in this regard, in-migration is the main cause of higher growth of population in most urban agglomerations, and particularly in Bangalore. On the other hand, low socio-economic development and consequent higher fertility is the major factor behind the higher population size and growth in Gulbarga district. The higher population size and growth in Belgaum district could be partly due to its proximity to Mumbai and its business impact stemming from social and economic backwardness of the district have led to higher population.

The growth rate of population in the decade 1991–2001 was higher in Bangalore (35%) and in most northern districts, i.e., Koppal (25%), Aichur (22%), Gulbarga (21%), Bidar (20%), Bagalkot (19%), Bijapur (18%) and Belgaum (17%). The reasons for higher growth of population in these districts are varied. While urbanization, industrialization, establishment of educational infrastructure, real-estate development, information technology and bio-technology ventures, etc., are held responsible for higher growth of population in Bangalore, demographic factors of high birth rates, fertility and regional inequality in socio-economic development are found responsible for the higher growth in population in the northern districts of Karnataka. The remaining districts of Karnataka witnessed medium rates in their size and growth in the decade under review. In contrast, the coastal district of Udupi and districts in the southern districts like Kodagu, Hassan and Mandya have witnessed low population growth rates (see Figure 3.3).

Figure 3.3
Districtwise Decadal Growth of Population in Karnataka

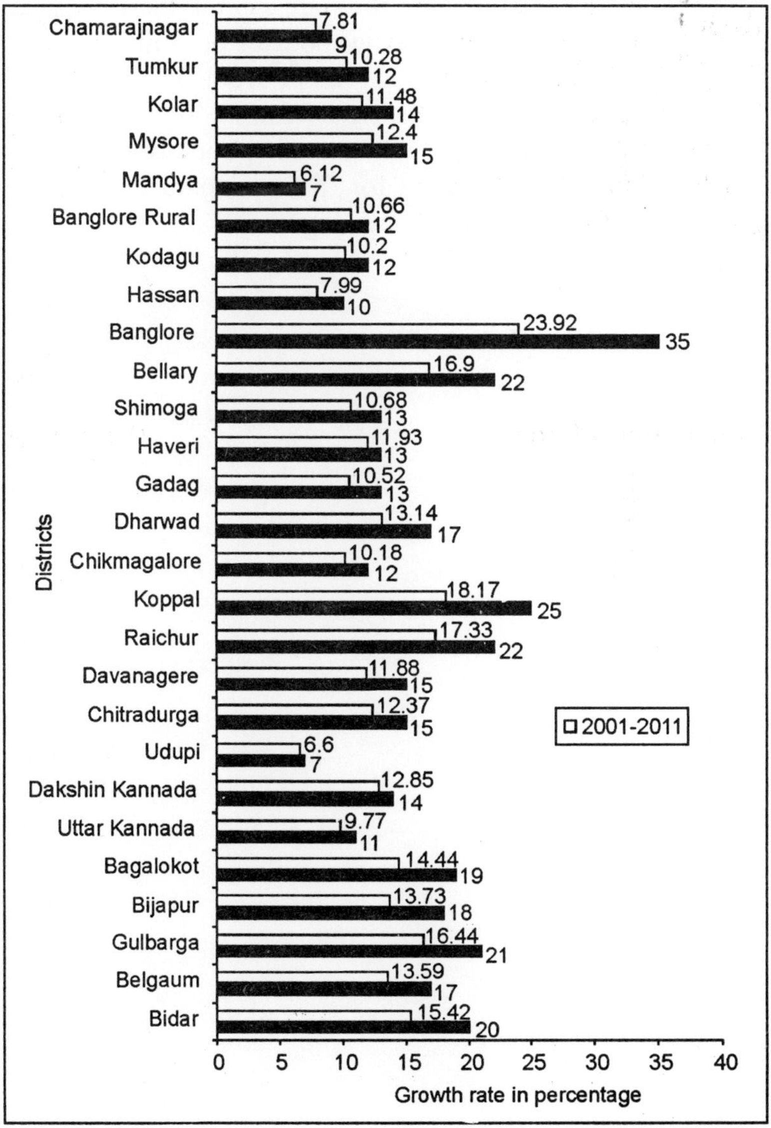

In the decade 2001–2011, the pattern of population growth across districts is more or less uniform in the state. Expectedly, growth rate has been coming down over time. Even in the case of Bangalore, the state capital, there has been a decline in population growth by about 11 percentage points, i.e., to 23.92 per cent in 2001–2011 from 35 per cent in 1991–2001. Similarly, all districts witnessed a more or less uniform trend in their growth rates of population, but the northern districts stands out for their comparatively higher rate of growth of population (see Figure 3.3).

4

Population Change in Karnataka

Distribution of population, as an aspect of population change, has gained importance over the years. In a developing country like India and particularly for a progressive state like Karnataka, population explosion is one of the important obstacles to economic development. However, population of a given area or a region is a resource for any kind of development.

In the last two decades of 20th century, globalization and other socio-economic developmental aspects have exerted influence on the growth of population. In certain regions characterized by metropolitan type of urbanization, migration had played a pivotal role in the growth and distribution of population. Viewed from this angle even micro-level studies at taluk level assume importance. Over the years, state and districtwise studies of population have become common. Several studies in Karnataka by both census organizations and researchers seem to share the same focus. The current study is specially focused on talukwise growth and distribution of population in 164 out of 175 taluks in Karnataka for the last two decades of 1981–1991 and 1991–2001. Further, a special investigation has been drawn to identify the social and economic causes for the differing patterns of population change in Karnataka by taluks.

In decade 1981–1991, Athani taluk of in Belgaum district recorded the maximum rate (86.24%) of population growth and in terms of growth rate it ranked first in the state. This was followed by Kustagi (27.92%), H.B. Hally (26.82%), Manvi (25.24%), Bidar (25.21%), Bhatkal (24.90), Raibagh (24.73), Kudligi (24.51%), Mysore (24.51%), Raichur (23.65%) and Lingasugur (23.63%) in their respective districts of Raichur, Bellary, Uttar Kannada, Belgaum and Mysore (see Annexure 1).

Taluks of Virajpet (–1.02) in Kodagu, Hosangar (1.37) and Thirthahally (4.68) in Shimoga, Sringeri (4.95) and Koppa (6.10) in Chickmagalur, Udupi (7.13) in Udupi, Kundgol (7.57) in Dharwad, Madikeri (7.61) in Kodagu district rank in descending order in the group of low growth rate taluks in the state. Likewise the taluks of Haliyal and Supa in Uttar Kannada district rank last in the state with negative population growth (–40.47 and –11.53).

These ranks of taluks based on population growth rates was much different in the decade 1991–2001, from the preceding decade. Due to rapid urbanization spurred by trade and commerce activities in Mangalore taluk in Dakshin Kannada district the rate of population growth was higher (23.96%). This was followed by Gulbarga, Gangavathi, Sindhanoor, Bellary, Kustagi, Devadurga, Mudhol, Koppal and Jevargi taluks respectively (see Annexure 1).

The average growth rate of population in Karnataka in the decade 1981–1991 was 21 per cent. The majority (88%) of the taluks recorded the growth rate below the state average, while only about 12.19 per cent of taluks had shown above the state average rate of population growth. This is because of the growth of industries, development of agriculture and other socio-economic infrastructure in the taluks that have helped greatly to achieve growth rates below the state average.

This distribution of population was almost same in the decade 1991–2001. Barely 2.44 per cent more taluks were added to the list of above state average growth rate taluks in the decade 1991–2001 making a total of 15 per cent compared with the decade 1981–1991. The rest, 85 per cent of taluks in the state remained below state average growth rate in population. There was slight reduction in the number of taluks below state average growth rate in the decade 1991–2001, consequent on the addition of taluks like Kolar, Bagalkot, and Mangalore to the group that had moved to higher growth rate bracket. Further, some taluks like Gulbarga, Gangavathi, Sindhanur, Bellary, Devadurga etc., had registered higher population growth in the decade 1991–2001.

The coefficient of rank correlation between the rate of population growth in 1981–1991 and 1991–2001 was found to be only 0.37, which is hardly significant at 0.01 levels. It is interesting to note that in the decade 1981–1991, about 6.70 per cent of the taluks had medium level of population growth, but this percentage went up to 24 per cent by the decade 1991–2001 (Figure 4.1).

Figure 4.1

Population Growth by Taluks in Karnataka

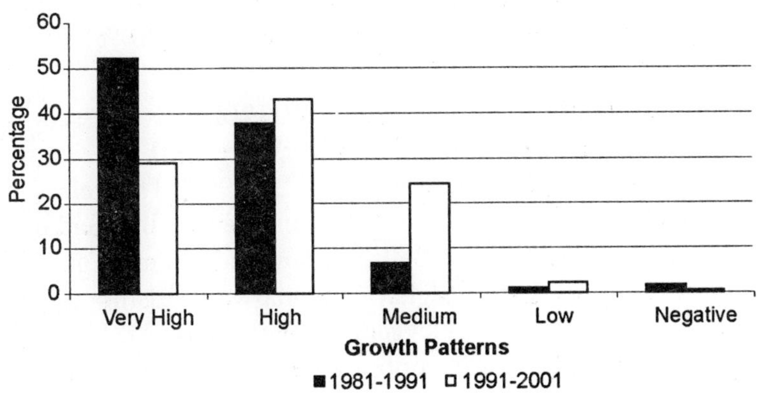

The mean and standard deviation of growth rate of population was lower at 12.35 and 5.68 respectively in the decade 1991–2001 as compared to figures of the preceding decade, i.e., 15.50 and 8.84 respectively. Development of modern agriculture and rural to rural migration had greatly influenced the substantial growth of rural population in the state.

Trends and Levels of Population Growth by Taluks

The present chapter briefly explains the overall scenario of population growth in Karnataka by taluks between 1981–1991 and 1991–2001. To understand the patterns of population growth in Karnataka by taluks, the growth rates have been classified into five groups: Very high rate of growth (VH), High (H), Medium (M), Low (L), and Negative (N). Figure 4.1 reveals that 86 (52.43%) out of 164 taluks in Karnataka, showed VH growth rate and 62 (37.80%) H growth rate in the decade 1981–1991. About 11 (6.70%) taluks had medium and negligible taluks, i.e., 2 and 3 taluks had low and negative level of growth rates respectively.

This distribution was significant in the decade 1991–2001 as compared to the previous decade, with virtual decline in number of VH taluks from 86 (52.43%) to 48 (29.26%). Further, there was also a marginal increase in the number of H level taluks from 62 (37.80%) to 71 (43.29%).

Significantly, the decade 1991–2001 witnessed a massive increase in the number of M level growth rate taluks in Karnataka from 11 (6.70%) to 40 (24.39%). This refers to the decline in growth rate of population in taluks like Badami, in Bagalkot, Hadagali in Bellary, Parasgad, Ramdurga and Sampagon in Belgaum, Kalghatgi in Dharwad, Krishnarajpete (K.R. Pete) in Mandya, Heggadadevanakote (H.D. Kote) in Mysore districts. It is noteworthy that, there was a remarkable decrease of VH level growth rate taluks (from 52.43 to 29.26%) in the decade 1991–2001, as compared to the preceding decade. Around 23 (52.43%) VH taluks reduced their growth rate from VH to H level by the decade 1991–2001. This is mainly an account of two significant factors: (i) declining birth rate from 27.6 in 1981 to 22 in 2001, low infant mortality (from 69 in 1981 to 58 in 2001) and (ii) rate of decline in fertility (from 3.5 in 1981 to 2.4 in 2001). Over the years, the efforts made by the Department of Health and Family Welfare in Karnataka through policies and programmes like sterilizations and IUD insertions have been remarkably successful in controlling people's participation in government initiatives; besides, higher levels of literacy had contributed to the reduction in population growth.

In this regard Table 4.1 presents the progress in family planning in Karnataka and how its helped in reducing population growth in Karnataka. It is evident that the progress achieved in sterilizations and IUD insertions in the state had pushed up cumulative number of sterilizations from 1.89 lakh in 1981–82 to 62.23 lakh in 1991–2001 and that of IUD insertions from 0.55 lakh in 1981–82 to 46.23 lakh in 1991–2001.

Further, the total number of sterilizations per 10,000 population in the age group 15–49 increased from 106 in 1981 and to 2,194 in 2001. Similarly, IUD insertions also increased to 3,339 in 2001 from 1505 in 1991 per 10,000 married women in the age group 15–49. This was sufficient proof for the success of health and family welfare programmes in Karnataka in controlling population growth.

Apart from this, it is also evident from Table 4.2 that, the overall social and economic development in the state, had to a great extent helped to bring down the rate of population growth rates during the decade between 1981–1991 and 1991–2001.

Table 4.1

Progress of Family Planning in Karnataka

Programmes	*1981–82*	*1991–1992*	*2001–2002*
No. of sterilizations*	1,89,000 (106)	28,05,600 (1241)	62,23,600 (2194)
IUD insertions*	55,000 —	16,58,700 (1505)	46,23,700 (3339)
Expenditure on public health in 9th Plan (Rs in lakh)	14478[a]	21914[b]	22909[c]

Source: Statistical Abstract India (1991 and 2002).

Notes: *Cumulative, a. 1996–1997, b. 1997–1998, c. 1998–1999. Parentheses indicates number of sterilizations per 10,000 population under age 15–49, and IUD insertions per 10,000 married women under age 15–49.

Table 4.2

Select Indicators of Demographic Social and Economic Development in Karnataka for the Year 1981, 1991 and 2001

Indicators	*1981*	*1991*	*2001*
Population Growth Rates	26.75	21.12	17.25
Crude Birth Rate	32.20	28.00	26.00
Infant Mortality Rate	69	77	58
Total Fertility Rate	3.5	3.1	2.4
Average Literacy	38.46	56.04	67.04
Female Literacy	27.71	44.34	57.45
Percentage of net area irrigated to net area sown	13.8	20.4	25.39
Percentage of urban population to total population	28.89	30.92	44.00
No. of employees per registered factories	55	102	96
Literacy (Total Female)	31.05	47.69	59.68
(a) Rural Female	19.77	34.76	48.50
(b) Total Rural	31.05	47.69	59.68

Source: Karnataka Socio-Economic Indicators 2002, Directorate of Economics and Statistics, Bangalore.

Note: *Refers to decadal growth rate as 1971–1981, 1981–1991 and 1991–2001.

Regionwise Population Growth in Karnataka

Geographically, Karnataka has been divided into three natural regions as Eastern Maidan, Malnad (Western Ghat) and Coastal Karnataka. The eastern region has been further divided into Northern and Southern Maidan regions. The northern region is drained by the Krishna, the Bheema and the Thungabadra river systems.

The districts of Bidar, Bijapur, Gulbarga, Bagalkot, Belgaum, Raichur, Dharwad, Koppal, Gadag, Haveri, Davanagere and Bellary come under northern region. Of the 175 taluks under 12 districts in Karnataka, 75 taluks in 12 districts come under northern region. This region covers 49.19 per cent of state's geographical area and holds 43.54 per cent of the state's population, registering a higher population density than other regions.

The southern region consists of nine districts, i.e., Chitradurga, Tumkur, Kolar, Bangalore (R), Bangalore (U), Hassan, Mandya, Mysore and Chamarajnagar and contains 64 taluks covering 30.73 per cent of geographical area and 41.86 per cent of population of the state (see Table 4.3).

The Malnad region consists of three districts, viz., Chickmagalur, Shimoga and Kodagu and includes 17 taluks, covering 10.30 per cent geographical area and 6.30 per cent of population of the state. Some parts of Hassan, Mysore, Dharwad and Belgaum districts also come under this region geographically.

The three districts of Uttar Kannada, Dakshin Kannada and Udupi consisting of 19 taluks comprises the coastal region; it covers 9.76 per cent of the state's geographical area and 8.26 per cent of population. The average normal rainfall is higher (3643 mm) in the coastal region and lowest (683 mm) in northern region. The southern (772 mm) and Malnad regions (2102 mm) comes next in order in the matter of average rainfall in the state.

Regionwise Population Change by Taluks

Table 4.4 gives the growth rates of population in 164 taluks of Karnataka contained in its four natural geographical regions. In the decade 1981–1991, 60 (80%) out of 75 taluks in northern region had recorded very high (VH) growth rates. What is noticeable here is that it is proved that population growth was slower in plains and hilly regions as compared to dry regions (Mehta, 1970). This is true in case of Karnataka, which consistently showed higher rates of population growth in dry region. With characteristic of high fertility and low mortality, population growth was quite high in the northern region. It is natural, therefore that Malnad region covering only two taluks registered VH level growth rate of population.

The southern and coastal regions occupies second (35.84%) and third (26.31%) positions respectively for having higher number of VH level taluks in the region. Here one could remember that, the study analysis excludes Bangalore and its urban district.

Most of the districts in northern region were identified as high fertility districts (NFHS II and III) in Karnataka, and in terms of socio-economic development, majority of the taluks were classified either as most or more backward taluks (Nanjundappa, 2002) in the state. No surprise therefore that 80 per cent of taluks in total taluks in the northern region had registered VH level growth rate.

Despite the above handicaps, crude birth rate declined from 32.2 in 1974–1981 to 28 in 1984–1990. This decline in population growth was the result of the initiatives taken by the Department of Health and Family Welfare in Karnataka as has been already referred. However, the districts which come under Hyderabad-Karnataka region, showed High (H) growth rate of population in the decade 1991–2001. Over the years the number of VH taluks have decreased to 37 (49.33%) from 60 (80%) in the region.

Table 4.3

Regionwise Area and Population

Region	*Administrative districts*	*Taluks*	*%age of area to total geographical area*	*Average %age of area to total geographical area of each district*	*%age of population to total population*	*Average %age of population to total population for each district*
Northern	12 (44)	75 (43)	49.19	4.09	43.54	3.62
Southern	9 (33)	64 (36)	30.73	3.41	41.86	4.65
Malnad	3 (11)	17 (10)	10.30	3.43	6.30	2.1
Coastal	3 (11)	19 (11)	9.76	3.25	8.26	2.75
Karnataka	**27 (100)**	**175 (100)**	—	—	—	—

Source: Karnataka at a Glance 2001–2002.

Note: Figures in parentheses are percentage of the total.

Also in the decade 1991–2001, number of VH taluks decreased from 35.84 to 15.09 per cent in southern region. The decline was from 26.31 per cent in 1981 to 10.52 per cent in 1991 in the case of the coastal region (see Table 4.4).

Globalization and other socio-economic developments of the 1990s have had its influence on the growth and distribution of population; the entire scenario changed in the decade 1991–2001, as contrasted with the previous decade. In both the decades, the VH taluks were found distributed in all the regions. Yet, there was a remarkable decrease in VH and H level taluks by the decade 1991–2001.

Under this population growth scenario, a notable feature is that, there was a remarkable decrease in the number of VH taluks even in the northern region which is still rather backward. On the other hand H level taluks increased to 46.66 from 18.66 per cent. Alongside the noticeable reduction in VH taluks in all the regions in the state, the share of H level taluks increased from 6.7 to 24.39 per cent in the decade 1991–2001. But, it should be borne in mind that growth rate figures of Karnataka in its sub-regions were lower than the national average growth rate and in almost all cases below the state figures too.

Districtwise Population Change by Taluks

It is evident from Table 4.5 that, there were no VH taluks in districts like Chickmagalur, Kodagu, Udupi and Chamaraj Nagar in the decade 1981–1991. The rest of the districts indeed had VH level growth rate taluks. If we look at the percentage of taluks in total taluks of a district, it is 80 to 100 per cent in Bijapur, Mysore, Raichur, Koppal, Gulbarga, Bellary, Haveri and Bidar districts. The reason behind this has been examined in the earlier section. Percentages of taluks in total taluks of the district were about 20 per cent in Tumkur and Gadag and 14.28 per cent in Mandya districts.

Table 4.4

Regionwise Population Growth by Taluks in Karnataka for the Decade 1981–1991 and 1991–2001

Region	*Decade 1981–1991*										*Decade 1991–2001*									
	Population growth patterns																			
	VH	%	H	%	M	%	L	%	N	%	VH	%	H	%	M	%	L	%	N	%
	Taluks																			
Northern region (75)	60	80.00	14	18.66	1	1.33	—	—	—	—	37	49.33	35	46.66	3	4.00	—	—	—	—
Southern region (53)*	19	35.84	33	62.26	1	1.9	—	—	—	—	8	15.09	18	33.96	25	47.16	2	3.77	—	—
Malnad region (17)	2	11.8	7	41.17	5	29.41	2	11.76	1	5.88	1	5.88	10	58.82	5	29.41	1	5.88	—	—
Coastal region (19)	5	26.31	8	42.10	4	21.05	—	—	2	10.52	2	10.52	8	42.10	7	36.84	1	5.26	1	5.26
Karnataka (164)	**86**	**52.4**	**62**	**37.8**	**11**	**6.7**	**2**	**1.21**	**3**	**1.82**	**48**	**29.26**	**71**	**43.29**	**40**	**24.39**	**4**	**2.43**	**1**	**0.6**

Source: Calculated from Table 1.
Note: Percentage calculated for the total taluks in a region
*Southern region excludes Bangalore urban and rural districts.

This growth rate pattern is a notable feature of the decade 1991–2001, which showed a clear reduction in VH taluks and increase in the number of H growth rate taluks. Excepting Raichur and Koppal, there were no other districts that had 100 per cent of its taluks under VH level of growth rates during the decade. Another noteworthy feature is the remarkable increase of medium (M) level taluks in this decade, as compared to the previous decade. Though there was a marginal increase in the number of H level taluks from 37.80 to 43.29 per cent of the total (see Table 4.5).

Major Changes in Patterns of Population Growth by Taluks

The earlier section contained a detailed investigation on the different patterns of population change across taluks in Karnataka. In this section an endeavour has been made to trace the major changes in the growth rates pattern of population in all the 164 taluks of Karnataka between the decade 1981–1991 and 1991–2001.

In the decade 1981–1991, 86 (52.43%) out of 164 taluks in the state recorded VH level growth rates (Annexure 4), but by the next decade, number of VH level growth rate taluks came down to 48 with 29.26 per cent (Annexure 6). For a close scrutiny of the growth rates of population, the VH taluks (86) have been divided into three groups: (i) taluks which demoted in their growth rate from VH to H and M level, (ii) taluks that remained in the same level, and (iii) taluks that moved up the ladder of growth rate from below (H, M, and L) to higher (VH) level.

Accordingly, 41 (47.67%) of the total (86) taluks come down from VH level to H level growth rate (Annexure 5) and a few other taluks, namely Hirekerur in Haveri district, Arkalgud and Holenarasipura taluks in Hassan district were demoted to M level from VH level by the decade 1991–2001.

Table 4.5

Districtwise Population Growth by Taluks in Karnataka for the Decade 1981–1991 and 1991–2001

District	***Decade 1981–1991***					***Decade 1991–2001***				
	Population growth patterns									
	VH	H	M	L	N	VH	H	M	L	N
	Taluks and Per cent of Taluks in total Taluks in district									
Chitradurga (6)	3 (50%)	3(50)				2(33.33)	2(33.33)	2(33.33)		
Davanagere (6)	4(66.66)	2(33.33)					6(100)			
Kolar (11)	4(36.36)	7(63.63)				2(18.18)	8(72.72)	1(9.09)		
Shimoga (7)	2(28.57)	2(28.57)	1(14.28)	2(28.57)		1(14.28)	4(57.14)	1(14.28)	1(14.28)	
Tumkur(10)	2(20)	8(80)				2(20)	3(30)	4(40)	1(10)	
Belgaum (10)	7(70)	3(30)				4(40)	6(60)			
Bijapur (5)	4(80)	1(20)				2(40)	3(60)			
Bagalkot (6)	4(66.66)	2(33.33)				4(66.66)	2(33.33)			
Dharwad (5)	2(40)	2(40)	1(20)				4(80)	1(20)		
Gadag (5)	1(20)	4(80)					4(80)	1(20)		
Haveri (7)	7(100)						6(85.71)	1(14.28)		

Cont'd...

Cont'd...

Uttara Kannada (11)	2(18.18)	5(45.45)	2(18.18)		2(18.18)	1(9.09)	4(36.36)	5(45.45)	1(9.09)	
Bellary (7)	7(100)					6(85.71)	1(14.28)			
Bidar (5)	5(100)					3(60)	2(40)			
Gulbarga (10)	10(100)					9(90)	1(10)			
Raichur (6)	6(100)					6(100)				
Koppal (3)	3(100)					3(100)				
Chickmagalur (7)		4(57.14)	3(42.85)				3(42.85)	4(57.14)		
Dakshin Kannada (5)	3(60)	2(40)				1(20)	4(80)			
Udupi (3)		1(33.33)	2(66.66)					2(66.66)		1(33.33)
Hassan (8)	3(37.5)	4(50)	1(12.5)				1(12.50)	7(87.5)		
Kodagu (3)		1(33.33)	1(33.33)		1(33.33)		3(100)			
Mandya (7)	1(14.28)	6(85.71)					1(14.28)	5(71.42)	1(14.28)	
Mysore (7)	6(85.71)	1(14.28)				2(28.57)	3(42.85)	2(28.57)		
Chamarajnagar (4)		4(100)						4(100)		
Karnataka (164)	**86(52.43)**	**62(37.80)**	**11(6.70)**	**2(1.21)**	**3(1.82)**	**48(29.26)**	**71(43.29)**	**40(24.39)**	**4(2.43)**	**1(0.60)**

Source: Calculated from Table 1.

45 taluks (52.32%) out of the remaining 86 continued as VH level taluks (Annexure 6).

In the earlier chapter we have already examined, to some extent, aspects like cumulative number of sterilizations and IUD insertions done in the last two decades. The significant progress achieved in health and family welfare measures in Karnataka as well as in the country as a whole has in no small measure influenced the overall growth rate of population in Karnataka and in reducing VH level growth and to the remarkable increase in medium level taluks. In this view it has witnessed that over the years, the health and family welfare programmes which were initiated by the governments have influenced to the downward trend in the growth rate of population.

Hirekerur taluk in Haveri district, Arkalgud and Holenarasipura taluks in Hassan district moved directly from VH level growth rate to M level. This is apparently due to the special features in the health and family welfare programmes here as also the success achieved in several other spheres of socio-economic development in the taluks.

Further investigation into the reasons for VH level growth rates in 48 taluks revealed the influence of mixed factors like demographic, social and economic causes as also the succors of health and family welfare programmes in Karnataka as the prime reason for changes in the growth rates of population in the study period.

Bijapur, Bagalkot, Bellary, Bidar, Gulbarga, Raichur and Koppal were identified as high fertility (NFHS II) districts. The major reason for VH level growth rate in these districts was higher fertility (NFHS II) and relatively low level of socio-economic development. It is to be borne in mind that lower the socio-economic development status, higher is the fertility and vice versa. Further, it is to be noted that these (33) taluks (except Bagalkot, Bellary and Gulbarga) identified as most and more backward taluks according to the Comprehensive Composite Development Index (CCDI) as reported by the eminent economist Nanjundappa (2002). The other reasons such as higher proportion of SC/STs and Muslims, urbanization, industrialization etc., were found to be responsible for VH level growth rate in rest of the 15 taluks, in the districts of Chitradurga, Kolar, Shimoga, Tumkur, Belgaum, Uttar Kannada, Dakshin Kannada, and Mysore.

It is assumed that higher the proportion of SC/STs and Muslims in total population of the district in a given region, higher is the fertility. Conversely, lower the proportion of above cited groups, lower the fertility. Challakere and Molakalmur taluks have higher percentage of ST population (35.23 and 15.79% respectively) as compared to other taluks in the district. These taluks also have low female literacy, besides falling under 'more' and 'most' backward taluks in CCDI. Challakere is known for agro-based industries and commercial trade while Molakalmur is famous for saree weaving manufacturing and household industries. The community-involved observation revealed that such manufacturing industries need to be more labour intensive. Traditional value system of the people might also have been responsible for high growth rate of population in spite of the birth control measures undertaken by the government.

Kolar taluk besides being the headquarters of the district, is also a centre of silk industry. It also has a higher concentration of SCs (10.92%) with over and about 23 per cent of families below poverty line. These were the causes for VH level population growth rates in Kolar taluk. Malur taluk shows signs of relative backwardness in comparison with taluks that have horticulture and sericulture. This explains the VH level growth in Malur taluk. Hence, it has shown VH level growth rate in the state.

Early arrival of agro-based industries and consequent development of economy in Shimoga district, is the cause for the VH level growth in the district. On the other hand Shimoga taluk alone has about 37.65 per cent of all registered industries and 42 per cent of urban population in the district total. The hypothesis number one has strongly proved that, owing to industrial development in taluks of southern region, particularly district of Shimoga taluk (district headquarters) has shown higher growth rates of population.

Tumkur taluk, the district headquarters of the district is the gateway to most of the northern districts in Karnataka. It is about 65 km away from Bangalore. Along NH 4, from Dabaspet to Chitradurga, there are found industrial establishments of different kind, i.e., small and medium scale metal, electronic and agro-based industries. Dahabas (roadside hotels), Automobile shops, petty shops etc. abound NH 4. The people who work in the units are mostly from neighbouring states like Kerala, Tamil Nadu, and Andhra Pradesh. The workers and owners, especially of Dahbas are from states like Punjab, Rajasthan etc.; and this has been causing migration. Another reason assumed for the sustained VH level growth of population in these two taluks was the comparatively higher percentage of Muslim population with its attendant high fertility.

What probably causes high level growth of population in taluks like Belgaum is the growth in and output from agriculture, coupled with the social and educational backwardness of the poorer sections that constitute the majority here. The taluks like Athani, Belgaum, Gokak and Raibagh in Belgaum district also showed VH level growth rate of population. Probably this was due to the agricultural incentives like expansion of irrigated area. For instance, the taluk of Raibagh, Gokak and Athani had higher percentage (86, 62 and 44% respectively) of irrigated area in total net sown area, than the other taluks in the district. Besides, about 15 per cent of SC population was found in Raibagh and 13 and 35 per cent of SC and ST population respectively was the cause for another reason for VH level population growth in Athani taluk. Surprisingly, it is to be noted that, one of the hypothesis which has been addressed in the study, that, higher the irrigated area represents the lower rate of population growth. In this view, it is reverse in case of the aforesaid taluks due to labour migration from neighbouring areas namely Raichur, Gulbarga into Bellary and Belgaum. Further, it seems to be higher growth rate of population.

There will be higher concentration of textile industries of the district total in taluk of Gokak (72%) leading to an influx of labour force from outside.

The above reasons were responsible for the VH level growth rate of population in Belgaum district. Belgaum being the headquarters of the district contains 66 per cent of all registered industries in the district. The urbanization and migration factors have had its influence on variation in growth of population. It is assumed that higher the irrigated area in the total cropped area of a given region, lower is the level of population growth and conversely lower the irrigated area higher is the level of population growth. Mandya district (down south) is a typical example. But Belgaum seems to be an exception to the rule in that despite the higher presence of SC/ST and poorer sections, population growth has been within norms.

With a larger proportion of rural population, and higher per cent of ST population and low female literacy, Mundgod taluk predictably has VH level growth rate of population in the district. This is in sharp contrast to the other taluks in Uttar Kannada district.

The VH level growth rate of population in Mangalore is not entirely due to higher births, but also due to industrialization and economic development. Besides development in trade and commerce, location of a large number of commercial banks (66.89%) of the district total, location of several educational and other allied activities all make Mangalore a hub of in-migration. Further, 84.54 per cent of Mangalore population is urban, and attracts migrants from other districts as well as from the neighbouring taluks in the state. Hence, factors related to economic, urbanization, industrialization, and migration were found responsible for this level of growth rate in Mangalore taluk.

People from other taluks of Mysore district have traditionally migrated to Mysore taluk. This is despite access to education through early opening of institutions, subsequent industrial development and emergence of other socio-economic activities like trade and commerce in almost all taluks of Mysore district. The significant size of tribal population, attendant backwardness and low literacy rates (as in H.D. Kote) is one of the reasons for VH level growth rate of population in Mysore taluk.

Comparatively, Piriyapatna taluk in Mysore district has more backward dry areas than other taluks. This will lead to poor socio-economic development. According to CCDI it is the most backward taluk in Mysore district. It is also true in case of Piriyapatna, the hypothesis has been listed relating to poverty and poor socio-economic status is determine the fact clearly.

With the reorganization process of City Municipal Councils in Karnataka, vide notification of 25 March 1998, 28 villages of Karkal taluk of Udupi district were transferred to Mangalore taluk of Dakshin Kannada district. This has resulted in the taluk of Karkal recording negative growth rate of population in the decade 1991–2001. This sort of reorganized process also may be the cause for negative growth rate of population in taluks of Haliyal and Supa in Uttar Kannada district in decade 1981–1991.

5

Rural Population Change

The total rural population of Karnataka in 1981 was 26 million; it increased to 31 million by 1991, and to 34 million by the year 2001. As mentioned in the previous chapter, the share of rural population in total population was found decreasing from 71 per cent in 1981 to 66 per cent in 2001. This decrease was mainly due to the rise in urban population during the last two decades in the state. Over the years, particularly after 1990s, globalization has to some extent influenced the distribution and growth of population in the state as well as in the country as a whole. Modern agriculture, industrialization, trade and commerce and such other activities in the region (Southern Maidan) contributed to rural-urban migration.

During the decade 1981–1991, the top ten taluks that recorded rural population growth in the state are: Athani (Belgaum), Mundgod (Uttar Kannada), Kudligi (Bellary), Sandur (Bellary), Kustagi (Koppal), Kalgatgi (Dharwad), Bhatkal (Uttar Kannada), H.B. Halli and Bellary (Bellary) and Bilgi in Bagalkot district. The bottom ten taluks are: Supa (Uttar Kannada), Udupi (Udupi), Mangalore (Dakshin Kannada), Virajpet (Kodagu), Hosanagar (Shimoga), Karwar (Uttar Kannada), Sakaleshpur (Hassan), Tirthahalli

(Shimoga), Yellapur (Uttar Kannada) and Sirsi in Uttar Kannada district (for ranks, see Annexure 2).

The expansion in irrigation, agriculture development and urbanization in the state had caused a rearrangement of existing ranking of taluks in terms of growth rate of rural population obtaining there by end of the decade 1991–2001. The taluks of Gangavathi (Raichur district) Koppal (Haveri district), Raibagh (Belgaum), Kustagi (Haveri), Sindanur (Raichur), Devadurga (Raichur), Mudhol (Bijapur), Bellary (Bellary), Lingasugur (Raichur) and Mangalore in Dakshin Kannada district had attained under top ten ranks in the state by the year 2001. On the other hand the taluks of Sandur in Bellary district has been pushed to the last rank in terms of the growth rate of population. Taluks of Karkal (Udupi), Ankola (Uttar Kannada), Kunigal (Tumkur), Sulya and Mundgod (Uttar Kannada) Chickmagalur in Dakshin Kannada district ranked behind Sandur in descending order.

The rural population in Karnataka decreased from 15 per cent in 1981–1991 to 10.75 per cent in 1991–2001. The mean growth rate of rural population was lowest in the decade 1991–2001, as compared to previous decade, as could be seen from the table below. There is a slight increase in standard deviation which reflects the substantial growth of rural population in the state during the decade 1991–2001.

Mean and standard deviation for growth rate of rural population for the decades 1981–1991 and 1991–2001 is as given below:

	1981–1991	*1991–2001*
Mean	15.34	9.72
Standard Deviation	8.72	9.61

The natural increase in the rural population, urbanization and rural to rural migration was the cause for lowest mean, and slight increase in standard deviation, in the growth rate of rural population in the state in decade under reference.

About 52.43 per cent of the 164 taluks in the state had growth rate below the state average in the decade 1981–1991. But, due to modern agriculture and impact of globalization on population growth and distribution and other tertiary functions, about 39.03 per cent of the taluks in rural Karnataka had recorded growth rates below the state average during the decade 1991–2001.

Trends and Levels in Rural Population Growth in Karnataka by Taluks

In the decade 1981–1991, about 83 per cent of the 164 taluks in Karnataka had VH and H level growth rates in their rural population, which come down to 72 per cent by the decade 1991–2001. At the same time, the number of medium level growth rate taluks increased to 26.21 per cent from 10.26 per cent by the decade 1991–2001.

It is clear that the declining birth rates (from 27.6 in 1981 to 24 in 2001) and as has been already mentioned in the previous chapter that, the significant progress achieved in the health and family welfare programmes, also had influenced the upward movement found in the medium level growth rate taluks, as opposed to the decreasing trend in VH level growth rate taluks in rural Karnataka.

Figure 5.1 reveals that 77 (46.95%) out of 164 taluks in the state registered VH level growth rate of rural population during the decade 1981–1991.

During the decade 1991–2001, there was a remarkable decrease in the number of VH level growth rate taluks in the state. The percentage decreased from 46.95 (1981–1991) to 18.9 (1991–2001). The number of medium level growth rate taluks increased from 10.36 to 26 per cent in this decade.

Figure 5.1
Rural Population Growth by Taluks in Karnataka

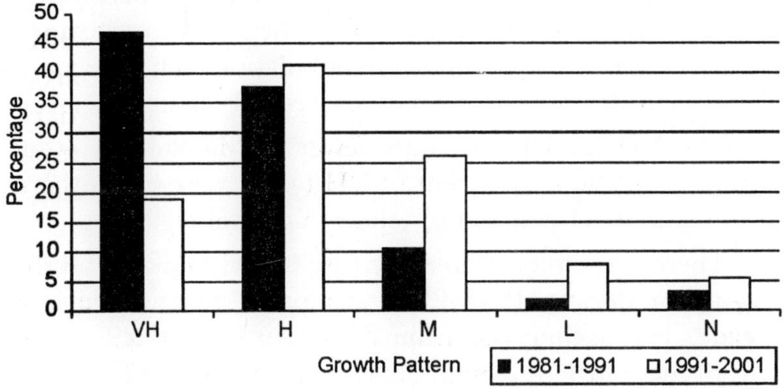

There was a marginal increase of H (high) level growth rate taluks in the state (i.e., from 37.8 to 41.46%).

As aforementioned in the previous chapter, the progress achieved in health and family welfare programmes and increasing literacy levels, particularly female literacy in rural Karnataka, were the major factors that have led to the creation of awareness in family planning etc., which in turn was responsible for virtual decline in the number of VH level growth rate taluks from 77 (46.95%) to 31 (18.9%) in the decade 1991–2001 (Table 5.1). At the same time it is interesting to note that, the efforts of the Department of Health and Family Welfare both at the state and central levels have been remarkably successful to motivate people to opt for smaller families. There were 18.9 per cent of taluks registered at VH level growth rate in rural population, in the decade 1991–2001 which testifies the fact that there has been perceptible development in the socio-economic status in Karnataka after globalization.

Region and Districtwise Rural Population Change in Karnataka

Of the four natural regions in Karnataka a higher percentage (74.66) of taluks of the district in northern region registered VH level growth rate in rural population. The frequent droughts in the state might have caused this change.

The VH level taluks were fewer in Malnad (11.76%) region, about 26.41 per cent of VH taluks were in southern region and 26.31 per cent of taluks in coastal region.

There was a remarkable decrease in VH taluks in all the regions in decade 1991–2001 compared to the previous decade. The decline was from 74.66 per cent to 29.33 per cent in the northern region, 26.41 per cent to 11.32 per cent in the southern region and 11.76 per cent to 5.88 per cent in Malnad region. In the coastal region this was from 26.31 to 10.52 per cent (see Table 5.1).

Growth rate figures of rural population by districts are given in Table 5.2. It is clear from the table that high fertility districts like Bellary, Bidar, Raichur, Koppal and Haveri had 100 per cent of its taluks in VH level growth rate group in the decade 1981–1991. District like Belgaum, Bijapur, Mysore, Gulbarga and Bagalkot were found to have 60 to 80 per cent of the total in the VH level growth rate group.

Table 5.2 further reveals that, the forest-based areas and industrially better placed districts of Shimoga, Uttar Kannada and Hassan have shown decline in the growth rates by the following decade, i.e. 1991–2001, the low level of growth in rural population had become more dispersed to cover the districts of Davanagere, Tumkur, Dharwad, Haveri, Chickmagalur and Mandya. Similarly parts of Shimoga, Uttar Kannada and Hassan districts also showed declining trends in population growth.

During the decade 1981–1991, districts of Chamarajnagar, Mandya, Gadag, Chitradurga, Kolar and

Tumkur had H level growth rate taluks. All the taluks of Chamarajnagar district showed H level growth rate, followed by Mandya (87.71%), Gadag (80%), Chitradurga (66.66%), Kolar (63.63%) and Tumkur (60%).

This situation was significantly different in the decade 1991–2001, from that of the previous decade; about 31 (18.90%) of the 164 taluks in the state had recorded VH level growth rate of rural population. The percentage being higher (46.95%) compared to the decade of 1981–1991. Interestingly, during the decade 1991–2001, excepting Raichur, there were no other districts in Karnataka with VH level growth rate in population. For further details see Table 5.2.

Major Changes in Rural Population Growth in Karnataka

Karnataka has a major share (66%, 2001) of rural population in its total population. However, Karnataka being a progressive state, of late, has come under the influence of globalization and urbanization as also modern technological development in agriculture. Consequently, such developments have started impacting the growth and distribution of rural population. This section, briefly examines the major changes in the growth rates of rural population in Karnataka.

During the decade 1981–1991, 77 out of 164 taluks in the state (46.95%) registered VH level of growth rate in their rural population (see Annexure 7). The number of VH level taluks declined to 31 (18.90%) by the decade 1991–2001. But, the decade also witnessed the inclusion of six new taluks in the group on their graduation from H to VH level growth rate. These taluks are Pavagada, Bagalkot, Sedam, Mangalore, Kundapur and Somavarpet.

For the detailed understanding of VH level growth rate taluks in the decade 1981–1991, they have been further

Table 5.1

Regionwise Rural Population Growth by Taluks in Karnataka for the Decade 1981–1991 and 1991–2001

Region	*Decade 1981–1991*										*Decade 1991–2001*									
	Population growth patterns																			
	VH	%	H	%	M	%	L	%	N	%	VH	%	H	%	M	%	L	%	N	%
	Taluks																			
Northern region (75)	56	74.66	17	22.66	2	2.66	—	—	—	—	22	29.33	40	53.33	7	9.33	4	5.33	2	2.66
Southern region (53)	14	26.41	32	60.37	6	11.32	1	1.88	—	—	6	11.32	17	32.07	24	45.28	5	9.43	1	1.88
Malnad region (17)	2	11.76	7	41.17	5	29.41	1	5.88	2	11.76	1	5.88	8	47.05	5	29.41	3	17.6	—	—
Coastal region (19)	5	26.31	6	31.57	4	21.05	1	5.26	3	15.78	2	10.52	3	15.78	7	36.84	1	5.26	6	31.57
Karnataka (164)	**77**	**46.95**	**62**	**37.8**	**17**	**10.36**	**3**	**1.82**	**5**	**3.04**	**31**	**18.9**	**68**	**41.46**	**43**	**26.21**	**13**	**7.92**	**9**	**5.48**

Source: Calculated from Annexure 2.
Note: Percentage calculated for the total taluks in a region.

Table 5.2

Districtwise Rural Population Growth by Taluks in Karnataka for the Decade 1981–1991 and 1991–2001

District	***Decade 1981–1991***					***Decade 1991–2001***				
	Population growth patterns									
	VH	H	M	L	N	VH	H	M	L	N
	Taluks and percentage of taluks in total taluks in district									
Chitradurga (6)	2(33.33)	4(66.66)				2(33.33)	2(33.33)	2(33.33)		
Davanagere (6)	3(50)	2(33.33)	1(16.66)				4(66.66)	1(16.66)	1(16.66)	
Kolar (11)	3(27.27)	7(63.63)	1(9.09)				8(72.72)	3(27.27)		
Shimoga (7)	2(28.57)	3(42.85)		1(14.28)	1(14.28)		4(57.14)	1(14.28)	2(28.57)	
Tumkur(10)	1(10)	6(60)	3(30)			1(10)	1(10)	6(60)	1(10)	1(10)
Belgaum (10)	6(60)	4(40)				3(30)	6(60)	1(10)		
Bijapur (5)	3(60)	2(40)					5(100)			
Bagalkot (6)	5(83.33)	1(16.66)				3(50)	2(33.33)	1(16.66)		
Dharwad (5)	2(40)	2(40)	1(20)				3(60)	1(20)	1(20)	
Gadag (5)	1(20)	4(80)					3(60)	2(40)		
Haveri (7)	7(100)						4(57.14)		2(28.57)	1(14.28)

Cont'd...

Cont'd...

Uttarakannada (11)	3(27.27)	4(36.36)	2(18.18)	1(9.09)	1(9.09)		2(18.18)	4(36.36)	1(9.09)	4(36.36)
Bellary (7)	7(100)					4(57.14)	2(28.57)			1(14.28)
Bidar (5)	5(100)					1(20)	4(80)			
Gulbarga (10)	8(80)	2(20)				3(30)	6(60)	1(10)		
Raichur (6)	6(100)					6(100)				
Koppal (3)	3(100)					2(66.66)	1(33.33)			
Chickmagalur (7)	–	3(42.85)	4(57.14)				3(42.85)	3(42.85)	1(14.28)	
Dakshin Kannada (5)	2(40)	1(20)	1(20)		1(20)	1(20)	1(20)	2(40)		1(20)
Udupi (3)		1(33.33)	1(33.33)		1(33.33)	1(33.33)		1(33.33)		1(33.33)
Hassan (8)	2(25)	3(37.5)	2(25)	1(12.5)			2(25)	5(62.5)	1(12.5)	
Kodagu (3)		1(33.33)	1(33.33)		1(33.33)	1(33.33)	1(33.33)	1(33.33)		
Mandya (7)	1(14.28)	6(85.71)					3(42.85)	2(28.57)	2(28.57)	
Mysore (7)	5(71.42)	2(28.57)				3(42.85)	1(14.28)	3(42.85)		
Chamarajnagar (4)		4(100)						3(75)	1(25)	
Karnataka (164)	**77(46.95)**	**62(37.80)**	**17(10.36)**	**3(1.82)**	**5(3.04)**	**31(18.90)**	**68(41.46)**	**43(26.21)**	**13(7.92)**	**9(5.48)**

Source: Calculated from Annexure 2.

subdivided into three groups: (1) taluks that demoted the growth rate from higher to lower positions (VH level to H, Medium and Low level) by the decade 1991–2001; (2) taluks which retained the same pattern (VH level) of growth rate, and (3) taluks that moved up in their growth rate from lower (H level) to higher (VH).

It is seen that of the 77, H level taluks, about 51 (66.23%) taluks moved to H, M or L level growth rates (see Annexure 9). Of this, H level growth rate taluks accounted for 65 per cent, followed by L (8%) and M (5%).

The urban population increased from 28 per cent (1981) to 34 per cent (2001). During the same period the growth rate of rural population in the state decreased from 17.66 to 12.05 per cent. In contrast, urban population remained largely the same; it went up from 29.62 per cent in 1981 to 28.85 per cent in 2001. As we have explained in the earlier section, the progress in health and family welfare programmes in the state have played a pivotal role in reducing VH level taluks in rural Karnataka from 77 (1981–1991) to 31 by the decade 1991–2001 (see Table 5.1).

In understanding the population growth and trends over the decades in the state we have tried to assign appropriate demographic, social and economic causes for the shift from VH to H, M and L levels.

Further, our investigation has been broadened to understand the causes for such changes in the growth rate of population.

During the decade 1991–2001, 21 out of 27 districts had experienced much reduced growth rate in their rural population in the state (see Annexure 9). As mentioned earlier, there were about 51 (66.23%) out of 77 taluks demoted in their growth rates from VH to H, M and L level. Declining fertility and awareness about family planning played an important role in reducing the rate of population growth in all over the state except some taluks of Bidar, Bellary, Bijapur, Gulbarga and Raichur districts. The districts of Haveri and Gulbarga, were having higher number of taluks in total taluks of the district. Hence, both demographic and migration factors were responsible for this change in the decade 1991–2001.

The level of urbanization was relatively high in southern districts like Davanagere, Kolar, Shimoga, Tumkur, Dharwad, Dakshin Kannada and Hassan. This could be the main reason for the decrease in numbers of taluks with higher growth rate in the above districts.

Districts of Belgaum, Bijapur, Bagalkot, Gadag, Haveri, Bellary, Bidar, Gulbarga, and Koppal had higher proportion of rural population in their total population. It is to be noted that due to development in modern agriculture the growth of urban population has been comparatively low in the taluks of these districts.

Over 25 (32.46%) taluks out of 77 recorded VH level growth rate in both the decades (see Annexure 10). Challakere and Molakalmur of Chitradurga district had higher rural population in their total population. The location of some rural household industry (weaving) in Molakalmur could be cited as the reason for this. Taluks of Athani, Gokak, and Raibagh in Belgaum district have higher area under irrigation as compared to other taluks in these districts, and this factor might have influenced the rural to rural migration. The substantial spread of irrigation in Bellary and Raichur districts could be cited as reasons for the large-scale migration from neighbouring districts into Bellary and Raichur (Sekher and Raju, 2000). Rest of the taluks in Bellary, Raichur, Koppal, and Mysore districts are equally ahead in terms of use of modern technology in agriculture and must have resulted in substantially higher concentration of rural population in these taluks during the decades under review.

A special investigation carried out in six taluks (Annexure 11) which moved up in their growth rates from H to VH level in decade 1991–2001, has thrown up interesting insights: Pavagada taluk in Tumkur district has a larger area under groundnut crop. The higher percentage of rural population in total population here is attributed to growth of agro-based industries dependent on groundnut cultivation, in the villages of Ponnasamudra, Mangalawada etc. Similarly, recent development in agriculture has raised Bagalkot taluk also into VH level growth rate. The situation is identical in Sedam and Kundapur taluks with relatively higher share of rural population compared to the position in the respective districts, i.e., Gulbarga and Udupi. Growth of plantation agriculture and resultant growth of rural population has pushed up the growth rates to VH level in Somavarpet taluk in Kodagu district.

6

Urban Population Change

The total urban population of Karnataka, in 1981, was 10 million. It increased to 13 million in 1991 and to 17 million by 2001. This is a rather rapid and continuous increase of urban population in the state. Industrial development is faster in southern region as compared to the other regions of the state. Growth of urban population was higher (59.14%) in the southern region. Employment opportunities, trade and commerce in districts of Bangalore, Mangalore, Mysore, Belgaum Dharwad etc., have attracted rural to urban migration to a great extent. Establishment of agro-based industries as also with information technology (IT)-related industries have been pulling population into urban areas. Over the years it became a characteristic factor of Southern and Coastal regions.

During the decade 1981–1991, the Athani taluk ranked first in the growth rate of urban population in the state. This is followed by Sedam (Gulbarga), Udupi (Udupi), Shahapur (Gulbarga), Sindanur (Raichur), Hosanagar (Shimoga), Bidar (Bidar), Tumkur (Tumkur), Puttur (Uttar Kannada), and Lingasugur (Raichur). On the other side, taluks of Kudligi (Bellary), Mudhol (Bijapur), Srirangapatna (Mandya), Hungund (Bagalokot), Sringeri (Chickmagalur), Haliyal (Uttar Kannada), Somavarpet (Kodagu), Chickmagalur

(Chickmagalur) and Aland (Gulbarga) came to occupy the last 10 ranks in the state in terms of population growth (see Annexure 3).

By the decade 1991–2001, the growth rate of urban population across taluks in Karnataka showed that the taluk of Kudligi in Bellary district ranked first in the state. This was followed by Shiggon (Haveri), Ankola (Uttar Kannada), Sindgi (Bijapur), Chickmagalur (Chickmagalur), the south-eastern parts taluks of Sidlagatta and Begepally (Kolar), Molakalmur (Chitradurga), Chicholli (Gulbarga) and Sira in Tumkur district.

The last 10 places in ranking in terms of low population were occupied by Kundapur (Udupi), H.D. Kote (Mysore), Karkal (Udupi), Hosanagar (Shimoga), Arkalgud (Hassan), Honnalli (Davanagere), Sandur (Bellary), Nagamangala (Mandya), Somavarpet (Kodagu) and Soraba (Shimoga) taluks.

Between the decades of 1981–1991 and 1991–2001, the urban population of Karnataka increased from 23.07 per cent to 23.52 per cent of the total. This increase is mainly due to the modernization in agricultural development in the state, especially estate agriculture in Malnad region, and increasing borewell irrigation from 9.36 per cent (1991) to 18.90 per cent (2001) resulting in to increased interaction (mobility) between urban and rural population.

Trends and Levels in Urban Population Growth in Karnataka by Taluks

Though the following table on talukwise growth of urban population shows a slight decrease in the growth rates, here one must bear in mind the rise in the absolute growth of urban population and that it varied across the state. Deliberately, the urban district of Bangalore metropolitan area and the rural district have been excluded from this analysis.

There was a marginal change in the growth rate of urban population across taluks between the decade 1981–1991 and 1991–2001. Table 6.1 gives the different patterns of urban population growth by taluks. In the decade 1981–1991, 99 (60.36%) out of 164 taluks recorded VH level growth rate. By 1991–2001, there was a marginal decrease in number of VH level taluks from 99 to 92. Likewise there was a downward shift in the number of H and L level growth rate taluks in the state.

Table 6.1
Urban Population Growth by Taluks in Karnataka for the Decade 1981–1991 and 1991–2001

Decade	*Population Growth Patterns*					
	VH	*H*	*M*	*L*	*N*	*Total*
			Taluks			
1981–1991	99	27	10	6	8	150*
%	60.36	16.46	6.09	3.65	4.87	100
1991–2001	92	23	15	3	17	150
%	56.09	14.02	9.14	1.82	10.36	100

Source: Calculated by the author.
*Data not available in 14 taluks (9 taluks in northern region and 5 in coastal region).

The growth rate below and above state average taluks was more generally identical in both the decades (68.66% in the decade 1981–1991 and 70% in 1991–2001).

Regionwise Urban Population Growth in Karnataka by Taluks

Ninety-nine (60.36%) out of 164 taluks in the state had very high (VH) level growth rate of urban population. The number of taluks in both northern and southern regions showing VH level growth rate of urban population was equal in the decade 1981–1991. Of this, if we look at the number of taluks in total taluks of each region was higher (81.13%) in southern region, and this is followed by northern (65.15%), coastal (57.14%) and Malnad region (29.41%). (For further details, see Table 6.2.)

It can be noticed that the early establishment of educational institutions and growth of power generation and industries in the southern region have led to higher growth of urban population. This has also resulted in a larger number of taluks in southern region recording VH level growth rates, in contrast to the other regions of the state.

In the northern region, on the other hand, a combination of a factors like demographic (high fertility), social and economic, including some kind of 'push' factor was found responsible for VH level of growth rate.

Belgaum city, the headquarters of Belgaum district has a large concentration of agro-industries, and several educational institutions (technical, medical and general). Similar institutions have also come up in Hubli, Dharwad, Gulbarga etc. National Highway 4 and major State Highways have remarkably upgraded their status and shape in recent years. This process is visible throughout the state, giving a fillip to the ongoing process of urbanization. In this, taluks of Hubli, Gulbarga, Athani, Belgaum etc., already have higher proportion of urban population.

A large chunk (21.42%) of H level growth rate of urban population taluks are found in the coastal region. This is followed by the northern, Malanad and southern region. Compared to the decade 1991–2001, there was a slight variation in the number of VH taluks in the state. However, there was no significant change in the position in the decade 1991–2001 (for details, see Table 6.2).

Table 6.2

Regionwise Urban Population Growth by Taluks in Karnataka for the Decade 1981–1991 and 1991–2001

Region	Decade 1981–1991										Decade 1991–2001								
	Population growth patterns																		
	Taluks																		
	VH	%	H	%	M	%	L	%	N	%	VH	%	H	%	M	%	L	%	N
Northern region (66)	43	65.15	13	19.69	2	3.03	4	6.06	4	6.06	49	74.24	10	15.15	5	7.57			2
Southern region (53)	43	81.13	8	15.09	1	1.88	_	_	1	1.88	32	60.37	7	13.2	6	11.32			8
Malnad region (17)	5	29.41	3	17.64	5	29.41	2	11.76	2	11.8	3	17.64	5	29.41	2	11.76	2	11.76	5
Coastal region (14)	8	57.14	3	21.42	2	14.28	_	_	1	7.14	8	57.14	1	7.14	2	14.28	1	7.14	2
Karnataka (164)*	**99**	**66**	**27**	**18**	**10**	**6.66**	**6**	**4**	**8**	**5.33**	**92**	**61.33**	**23**	**15.33**	**15**	**10**	**3**	**2**	**17**

Source: Calculated from Annexure 3.
Note: Percentage calculated for the total taluks in a region
*Data not available in 14 taluks (9 taluks in northern region and 5 in coastal region).

Major Changes in the Growth Rate Patterns of Urban Population in Karnataka

After 1990s there has been a remarkable growth in urban population in the state of Karnataka from 10.73 million in 1981 to 17.91 million in 2001. It is in variation from district to district and region to region. As mentioned above, relatively due to faster growth of industries, infrastructure development and urbanization southern region recorded higher growth rate of VH level taluks. Modern technological developments in agriculture and a variety of agro-based industries came into existence in many parts of the state, and this has led to higher growth of urban population in taluks like Chitradurga, Tumkur, Tiptur Gadag Athani etc. In this section, we examine the broad changes in the growth rate of urban population by taluks in the state.

During the decade 1981–1991, 99 out of 164 taluks in Karnataka registered VH level growth rates in their urban population. By the decade 1991–2001, there was a marginal decline in the number of taluks from 99 to 92 in this growth. Further, the taluks are classified into two major groups: (1) taluks which have been demoted in the growth rate from VH to H, M, L or negative by the decade 1991–2001, and (2) taluks which continued in VH level in both the decades.

As per this classification, there were 99 VH level taluks as of 1991 (see Annexure 12), 27 taluks (27%) which were demoted from VH to H level (see Annexure 13), with the rest of 73 per cent remaining in VH level as of 1991–2001(Annexure 14). Strangely, during the same period, about 20 new taluks moved on to VH level growth rate from H, M and L (see Annexure 15).

There has been a remarkable rise in infrastructure development like provision of drinking water, electricity, and road development in urban areas. The rural poor migrate to urban areas in search of livelihood/better living. Rural poverty, famine like conditions, particularly rising unemployment etc., are the causative factors for this incessant migration of rural youths to urban areas. Some of positive aspects of development like growth in sericulture, dairying etc., have to some extent checked mindless migration of people to urban areas. Availability of educational institutions in rural hinterland and better road transport have led to marginal decline in the exodus of rural folks to urban areas. For instance, there were 99 taluks (60.36%) under VH level growth rate in the decade 1981–1991; their number came down to 92 (56.09%) by the decade 1991–2001 (Table 6.1).

The other reasons responsible for decrease in the number of taluks with higher growth rate of urban population were the expansion of sericulture in the taluks of Chikkaballapura, Gouribidanur, and Gudibanda in Kolar district. Irrigation development in Hosanagar and Soraba taluks in Shimoga district, Hemavathi irrigation project to provide water for irrigation in Turvekere taluk of Tumkur district, development of plantation and other agriculture in Hassan, Uttar Kannada, Udupi and Mandya district etc., have helped to a great extent in bringing down the number of taluks from VH level growth rate to H and L levels.

It is difficult to unravel the reasons for the very high level of urbanization being confined only to certain areas of certain taluks. However, the continuous growth of urban population, high fertility (as in Gulbarga and Bagalkot), trade and commerce (as in Mangalore), educational infrastructure, employment opportunity provided by construction industry (both public and private sectors) in the districts of Mysore, Tumkur, Shimoga, etc., were some of the reasons for the continuation of about 72 taluks in VH level growth rate in the decade 1991–2001 and 1981–1991 (see Annexure 14).

The ongoing infrastructure development under the impact of globalization across the state may further accentuate the growth rates. It is hoped that rural development under "PURA" as envisaged by Dr A.P.J. Abdul Kalam, will further even out the growth rates both urban and rural. Spread of mass media particularly television to rural areas, from the 1990s has provided the needed push to urban and rural growth, particularly from 2001, and will continue to influence this process in the future also. Quality urbanization depends on the participation of minority communities, particularly in population control and other spheres of development without which reduction of in population growth would be difficult.

7

Changing Child Population in Karnataka

Over a period of two decades, there has been a continuous decrease of child population in the total population of Karnataka. This is the result of two demographic trends: first, the movement towards smaller families over the century meant fewer children were being born in the later part of the century; second, increase in life expectancy has led to a larger adult population in the recent decades. However, here one must note that declining fertility, increasing strong preference for male child in the modern society particularly in India, have further influence on unequal growth and distribution of male and female child population.

The proportion of youth, children and adults in the total population in a given region/area has played an important role in the socio-economic development and its growth. For instance, many developing economies like India, Pakistan, Africa and Sri Lanka have overexploited the available natural resources. This is because of higher proportion of child population in the total population. Despite this, it has led to low socio-economic development. Increasing awareness towards family planning in India since 1980s, contraception prevalence rate turned higher (59% Reproductive and Child

Health, Karnataka, 2002–2004). At the same time availability and access of health care services for children have also increased over time. This is true both for India and the progressive state of Karnataka. In this regard the Department of Health and Family Welfare, Government of India has made good effort in providing health care services and also controlling the population growth as well, by introducing innovative policies and programmes in the country. This is significant in Karnataka.

In this respect, the present section of the analysis deals with understanding the proportion of child population to total population and also to trace the major changes in its growth and distribution in Karnataka by districts for the decades 1981–1991 and 1991–2001. The first section briefly explains the proportion and growth of child population under age 0–6 in Karnataka. Further, an analysis has been done in understanding the demographic shift and its effect on the growth rate of child population under age 0–6 in Karnataka by districts over a period of time. A special emphasis has been laid to understand the growth rate of female child population in the context of increasing son preference and neglecting girl child in the modernizing society with increasing socio-economic development in Karnataka. A comparative analysis has been done for the last two decades for 1981–1991 and 1991–2001. The study also has certain the following assumptions:

1. Due to higher contraception prevalence rate, with low fertility and higher age at marriage in districts of southern region, there seems to be lower proportion of child population in the study period.
2. Availability of sophisticated health services by the public and private health institutions in southern districts of Karnataka has influenced the higher growth of male child population.

Change in Proportion: A Glance

Before understanding the growth, trends and levels of child population in Karnataka, it is necessary to mention the changes in proportion of child population under age of six years between 1981 and 2001. The child population of Karnataka increased from 6.84 million in 1981 to 7.47 million in 1991, but, by the year 2001 there was a decline in its absolute figures to 7.18 million. Figure 7.1 reveals that over the years the proportion of child population in total population has decreased from 18.4 per cent in 1981 to 13.6 per cent in 2001. This can be attributed to fall in fertility rates, birth rate and the increase in life expectancy (Table 7.1) has also influenced the reduction in the share of child population in total population of Karnataka.

Figure 7.2 presents the districtwise child population proportion for the year 1981, 1991 and 2001. There was a higher proportion of child population in Karnataka in all the districts in 1981 as compared to the year 2001. The average proportion of child population of the state in the year 1981 was 18.4 per cent. The districts of Bellary, Bidar, Bijapur, Chitradurga, Dharwad, Gulbarga, Kolar, Mandya and Raichur have registered above state average of 18.4 per cent. Whereas the other districts of Bangalore (U), Belgaum, Chickmagalur, Dakshin Kannada, Uttar Kannada, Tumkur, Hassan, Mysore, and Shimoga have shown below state average of child population in Karnataka.

As per 1991 Census, this proportion of child population in Karnataka declined slightly in all the districts except in Belgaum, Bidar, Gulbarga and Raichur. Interestingly, in the year 2001, there was a steady decline in the proportion of child population in all the districts in Karnataka.

For the purpose of understanding, the proportion of child population has been classified into four categories as high (18.1–22% or greater), medium (14.1–18%), low (10.1–14%) and very low (proportion below 10%). As per this classification, in the year 1981, the districts of Kodagu, Bangalore (U), Belgaum, Chickmagalur, Dakshin Kannada, Uttar Kannada, Tumkur, Hassan, Mysore and Shimoga are under medium (14.1–18%) category and the rest of the districts have come under high proportion category with 18.1–22 per cent in the total population. Interestingly it was clear from the Table 7.2 that there were no districts under the categories of low (10.1–14%) and very low (below 10%) in the year 1981. There was a wide variation in the child population proportion in 2001 as compared to the year of 1981. There were no districts under the categories of very low and high proportion child population. All the districts fall under low and medium proportion of child population.

Figure 7.1

Proportion of Child Population Under Age of 6 in the Total Population of Karnataka

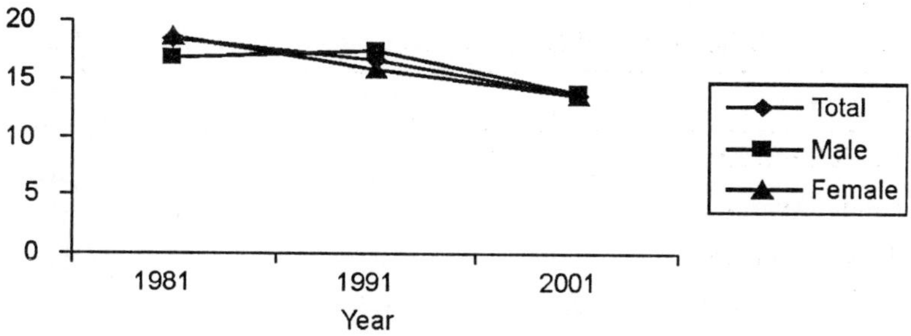

This was the significant change in the proportion of child population in Karnataka, over a period of time. With this evidence we could infer that demographic impact, as well as awareness of family planning and also, to some extent, improvement in socio-economic development have together attributed to low birth rates and intended fewer children in the last two decades.

Further it is clear from Table 7.2 that, the southern districts in Karnataka have been classified under low (10.1–14%) category, and rest of the districts in the northern region under medium category in proportion of child population. Though, studies have shown that this is because of two factors: (i) in Karnataka, especially most of the districts in northern region have registered high fertility, low age at marriage, and low female literacy (NFHS II and III), and (ii) comparatively low socio-economic development and the state has achieved expected demographic goals to a considerable extent. On the other hand, poverty reduction, fertility decline, increasing female literacy, reduction in infant and child mortality, availability and access of public health care services for children and particularly creating awareness about family planning programmes even in poorer and weaker sections of the society have influenced to a great extent in reducing child population in Karnataka in general and the southern districts in particular.

Table 7.1

Achievements of Demographic Goals in Karnataka

Indicators	*1981*	*1991*	*2001*
Crude Birth Rate	32.20	28	25
Crude Death Rate	—	8.1	7.6
Total Fertility Rate	3.5	3.1	2.4
Contraception Prevalence Rate	—	—	59.3*
Infant and Child Mortality Rate	69	77	58
Life Expectancy			
Total	—	61.9	63.3
Male	—	60.2	61.6
Female	—	63.5	64.9

Source: Population Change in Karnataka, Project Report submitted to ISEC by C.M. Lakshmana (2006) and * RCH Phase I &II, 2001, currently married women age 15–44.

Figure 7.2

Percentage of Child Population Under Age of 6 in Total Population of Karnataka by Districts

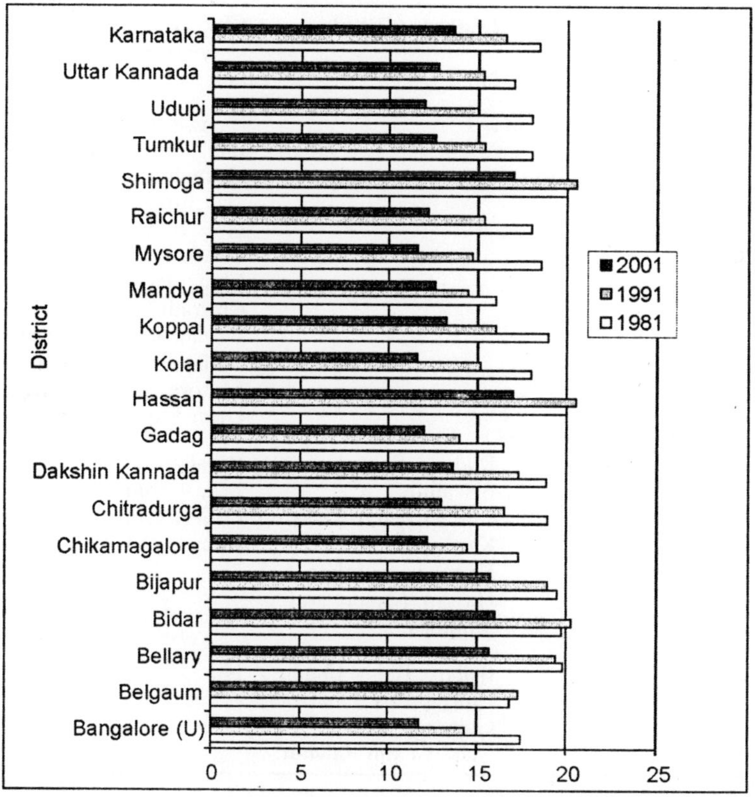

Proportion Change: Male-Female Child Population in the Total Child Population

In 1981 the proportion of male child population in total child population of Karnataka was 49.2 per cent; it increased to 53.4 per cent in 1991. But, there was a sharp decline of 51 per cent in its proportion in 2001. Interestingly, it is clear from the Table 7.3 that the proportion of female child population in the year 1981 was higher than that of male child population. But there was a noticeable change in its

Table 7.2

Proportion of Child Population Under Age of 6 years in Karnataka by District for the Year 1981 and 2001

Group	*Districts (1981)*	*(2001)*
Below 10% (Very Low)	Nil	Nil
10.1–14% (Low)	Nil	Bangalore (U), Bangalore Rural, Chamarajnagar, Dakshin Kannada, Hassan, Mandya, Tumkur, Udupi, Chickmagalur, Chitradurga, Davanagere, Dharwad, Gadag, Kolar, Kodagu, Mysore, Shimoga and Uttar Kannada.
14.1–18% (Medium)	Kodagu, Bangalore (U), Belgaum, Chickmagalur, Dakshin Kannada, Uttar Kannada, Tumkur, Hassan, Mysore and Shimoga.	Bagalkot, Belgaum, Bellary, Bidar, Bijapur, Haveri, Gulbarga, Koppal and Raichur.
18.1–22% (High)	Bellary, Bidar, Bijapur, Chitradurga, Dharwad, Gulbarga, Kolar, Mandya and Raichur.	Nil

Source: Compiled and classified by the author.

proportion in 1990. Increasing son preference, neglecting girl child and the increasing cost of education and marriage of girls etc., are the reasons for a sharp decline in the proportion of female child population. However, the proportion increased from 46.6 per cent in 1991 to 49 per cent in 2001. It shows that there has been a balanced growth of male/female population in Karnataka with the progressive status in the last decade of the 20th century. Of course, as has already been mentioned in the earlier part, increasing strong son preference, high cost involved in the marriage of girls are a major drain on the household resources, which also is a strong disincentive to have daughters (Sekher, 2006). This led to decreasing share of female child population in the total population of Karnataka. This also is true in the case of India. In Karnataka the female child population share was almost 51 per cent in 1981; it decreased to 46.6 per cent in 1991 but it further increased to 49 per cent in 2001.

Table 7.3

Proportion of Child Population (Male and Female) in Total Child Population in Karnataka by Districts

District	***For Males***					
	1981	***%****	***1991***	***%***	***2001***	***%***
Bangalore (U)	436839	50.4	355711	51.2	772540	51.4
Bangalore (R)	—	—	133378	51	225618	51.4
Bagalkot	—	—	—	—	264872	51.5
Belgaum	273351	50.8	316944	51.1	624031	52
Bellary	150330	51	187804	51	319086	51.3
Bidar	101851	51.5	130458	51	241517	51.5
Bijapur	238398	50.8	284405	51	286831	51.9
Chamarajnagar	—	—	—	—	114937	51
Chickmagalur	79404	50.4	74432	50.5	138644	51
Chitradurga	169247	50.2	362537	51	199535	51.3
Davanagere	—	—	—	—	240275	51.3
Dharwad	285333	_	311296	51.2	218262	51.4
Dakshin Kannada	199208	50.6	193036	50.8	228060	51.2
Gadag	—	—	—	—	137835	51.2
Gulbarga	211602	50.8	269659	51	536454	51.6
Haveri	—	—	—		203712	51
Hassan	122117	49.9	121120	50.8	199665	51

Cont'd...

Cont'd...

Kolar	179470	50	180627	50.7	336469	51
Koppal	—	—	—	—	208004	51.2
Kodagu	38602	50.7	36073	50.7	69574	50.5
Mandya	131324	49.9	123204	51	205147	51.6
Mysore	236666	50.7	247858	50.8	323555	51
Raichur	179522	50.5	240742	50.8	283068	50.9
Shimoga	150742	50.5	150434	50.9	208163	51
Tumkur	182715	50.9	177259	50.7	308162	51.2
Udupi	—	—	—	—	114581	51
Uttar Kannada	97314	51.3	96139	51.3	173503	51.3
Karnataka	3178702	49.2	3993116	53.4	7182100	51

District	***For Females***					
	1981	***%***	***1991***	***%***	***2001***	***%***
Bangalore (U)	429880	49.6	337912	48.8	374892	48.6
Bangalore (R)	—	—	—	49.0	109446	48.6
Bagalkot	—	—	—	—	128308	48.5
Belgaum	265117	49.2	302531	48.9	299215	48.0
Bellary	144625	49	179800	49.0	155194	48.7
Bidar	95804	48.5	125531	49.0	117116	48.5
Bijapur	231050	49.2	271791	49.0	138081	48.1
Chamarajnagar	—	—	—	—	56426	49.0
Chickmagalur	78121	49.6	72760	49.5	67865	49.0
Chitradurga	167616	49.8	177524	49.0	97023	48.7
Davanagere	—	—	—	—	116779	48.7
Dharwad	271041	_	296234	48.8	105927	48.6
Dakshin Kannada	194200	49.4	186417	49.2	111206	48.8
Gadag	—	—	—	—	67208	48.8
Gulbarga	204641	49.2	258689	49.0	259611	48.4
Haveri	—	—	—	—	99593	49.0
Hassan	122671	50.1	117177	49.2	97694	49.0
Kolar	179224	50	175464	49.3	164741	49.0

Cont'd...

Cont'd...

Koppal	—	—	—	—	101505	48.8
Kodagu	37550	49.3	36313	49.3	34382	49.5
Mandya	131655	50.1	118152	49.0	99089	48.4
Mysore	229817	49.3	239338	49.2	158621	49.0
Raichur	175669	49.5	232267	49.2	138971	49.1
Shimoga	147717	49.5	144609	49.1	101740	49.0
Tumkur	176265	49.1	171970	49.3	150083	48.8
Udupi	—	—	—	—	56072	49.0
Uttar Kannada	92233	48.7	91254	48.7	84354	48.7
Karnataka	3286570	50.8	3484495	46.6	3491142	49.0

Source: Censuses of India, 1981, 1991 and 2001.
Note: *Percentage to total Child Population under age 0–6.

It indicates that there had been an increasing share of female child population in Karnataka during the years between 1991 and 2001, with the increasing progress of socio-economic development. Hence, it is a satisfactory aspect and relatively better sign of gender equity in male dominated society in Indian states. Based on this the study concludes that development process in Karnataka is closely associated with gender equity. However, it varies across districts. This has been discussed in the next section.

Growth Rate Trends and Levels: Total Child Population

In the decade 1981–1991, the overall growth rate of child population in Karnataka was 8.5 per cent. But, it was negative in the decade 1991–2001. It can be seen from the Table 7.4 that in the decade 1981–1991 most of the northern districts like Belgaum, Bellary, Bidar, Bijapur, Chitraduraga Dharwad, Gulbarga, Raichur and the districts of Mysore, Dakshin Kannada in southern region had registered positive growth rates of child population in the state. But during the decade

Table 7.4
Decadal Growth of Child Population Under Age of 6 in Karnataka by Districts

District	*Decade*		*Per cent*
	1981–1991	*1991–2001*	*Increase or decrease*
Bangalore (U)	–25	10.2	35.2
Bangalore (R)		–15.7	
Bagalkot			
Belgaum	18.7	0.7	–18
Bellary	19.8	–15.2	–35
Bidar	22.8	–6	–28.8
Bijapur	15.6	–0.81	–16.41
Chamarajnagar			
Chickmagalur	–7	–6.2	0.8
Chitradurga	7.1	17.56	10.46
Davanagere			
Dharwad	8.4	–0.08	–8.48
Dakshin Kannada	3.7	–10.74	–14.4
Gadag			
Gulbarga	21.2	1.5	–19.7
Haveri			
Hassan	–2.7	–19.3	–16.6
Kolar	–0.7	–5.8	–5.1
Koppal			
Kodagu	–7.1	–2.2	4.9
Mandya	–9	–17.7	–8.7
Mysore	4.3	–11.10	–15.4
Raichur	24.9	3.67	–21.23
Shimoga	–1.2	–41.7	–40.5
Tumkur	–2.8	–13.3	–10.5
Udupi			
Uttar Kannada	–1.1	–8	–6.9
Karnataka	8.5	–4.1	–12.6

Note: Calculated by the author.

1991–2001, there had been a drastic change in the growth rate of child population across districts in Karnataka. Excepting the districts of Chitradurga, Bangalore Urban (10.2%), Belgaum (0.7) Gulbarga (1.5) and Raichur the rest of the districts had shown negative rate of growth in child population under age 6. In the decade 1981–1991 the districts like Belgaum, Bellary, Bidar and Bijapur had posted higher levels (15.1–20%) of growth in child population.

Economically backward districts of Gulbarga and Raichur had registered very high (20.1% or more) growth rates. It is observed that most of the districts in southern region like Bangalore Urban, Chickmagalur, Uttar Kannada, Hassan, Kolar, Kodagu, Mandya, Shimoga and Tumkur had registered negative rates of growth in child population in the state. Here one must note that the growth of child population was not only low, but also negative in the decade 1991–2001. Interestingly the districts of Chitradurga and Dharwad have shown low (5.1–10%) growth rates in their child population.

If we compare the growth rates of child population in decade 1991–2001 with that of 1981–1991, it shows that excepting Belgaum, Gulbarga (below 5%), and Bangalore Urban (10.1–15%) no other districts reported positive growth rates in child population in the state (Table 7.5). From this, we could infer that over the years the developing country of India experienced decline in fertility rates at the national level. However, there is a growing disparity between northern states and southern states with the southern states being more successful in controlling population growth (Gulimoto and Rajan 2005). Awareness about small family, welfare programmes and policies and increasing female literacy rate resulted in controlling population growth and has played an important role in reducing the growth rate of child population in Karnataka.

Table 7.5

Decadal Growth of Child Population Under Age of 6 in Karnataka by District for the Decade 1981–1991 and 1991–2001

Growth Rate Levels	*1981–1991 districts*	*1991–2001 districts*
Negative (less than 0%)	Bangalore (U), Chickmagalur, Uttar Kannada, Hassan, Kolar, Kodagu, Mandaya, Shimoga and Tumkur	Bangalore (R), Bellary, Bidar, Bijapur, Chickmagalur, Dharwad, Dakshin Kannada, Hassan, Kolar, Kodagu, Mandya, Mysore, Shimoga, Tumkur and Uttar Kannada
Very Low (below 5%)	Dakshin Kannada, Mysore	Belgaum, Gulbarga and Raichur
Low (5.1–10%)	Chitradurga, Dharwad	Nil
Medium (10.1–15%)	Nil	Bangalore (U)
High (15.1–20%)	Belgaum, Bellary, Bidar and Bijapur	Chitradurga
Very High (20.1% or greater)	Gulbarga and Raichur	Nil

Source: Classified by the author.

There were two reasons for positive (very low) growth of child population in districts of Bangalore Urban, Gulbarga and Belgaum. First, increasing slum population and rapid migration to Bangalore Urban district seem to have contributed to the positive growth of child population. Further investigation has been done on the aspects of geographical boundary of Bangalore (U). Both in 1991 and 2001 the geographical boundary was 2,190 sq km. Hence, it is clear that the higher growth of child population under age of 6 is not due to boundary change. The large proportion of labour migrants towards Belgaum from other parts of Karnataka in search of employment coupled with high fertility among migrant population seem to have higher growth of population. In this regard migration data from successive censuses indicate that about 87 per cent of the total migrants were recorded either inter-district or intra-district migrants within the state. Border districts like Bellary, Belgaum, Kodagu, Bidar and Kolar had a higher proportion of migrants from other states (Sekher, 2004). Secondly it is to be noted that poor economic position, illiteracy and also their religious way of life to some extent seem to be the main reasons for positive growth in child population in the district of Gulbarga. However, this calls for further research to unearth the exact reasons on this issue. However, here one must note that out of 640 towns in India, about 28 towns have 2 lakh and above slum population, with Bangalore being one of them. The remaining 612 towns out of 640 have 25,000 to 1 lakh slum population (Census of India, 2001, Series 1, Slum Population India). Illiteracy and low socio-economic status among the slum population might be the reason for the high growth of child population irrespective of the sex.

Growth Rate Trends and Levels: Male Child Population

It is a general phenomenon that historically the Indian society is a male dominant one along with gender discrimination. In view of this the proportion and growth of male child population in total population of a country/ region assumes greater importance in population studies. There have been many districtwise as well as statewise studies in India which focus on gender related issues. In this context if we examine the proportion and growth of gender based population under age of 6, one can observe that there has been a wide gap in the growth of male and female child population in Karnataka. It is a well-known fact that Karnataka of late is playing an important role not only as a progressive state but also in the economic development scenario of the country.

It is evident from Table 7.6 that the decadal growth of male child population under age six was 20.40 per cent in decade 1981–1991. But, it was absolutely negative in the next decade of 1991–2001. Hence, from this observation one can note that probably due to increasing awareness about family planning and the effort made by the Department of Health and Family Welfare in the country has influenced to a negative growth of child population with a declining trend (– 8.2%) in the decade 1991–2001.

If we look at the percentage change of male child population under age six between the two decades as reported from Table 7.6 that, except the districts of Bangalore (33.35%), Kodagu (4.51%) and Chickmagalur (1.52%) the rest of the districts were absolutely negative growth of child population in the state. In decade 1981–1991 the districts of Raichur (25.43%), Bidar (21.93%) and Gulbarga (21.43%) have registered above state average growth rate of 20.40 per cent. Even the district of Bellary (19.95%), Bijapur (16.18%) and Belgaum (13.75%) districts had also registered relatively higher growth of child population under age 6 in Karnataka. The minimum growth rate has been reported in districts of Kolar (0.64%), followed by Dharwad (8.34%) and Chitradurga (8.52%). The growth rate was negative in the remaining districts of Karnataka.

The above scenario has been entirely changed in decade 1991–2001 when compared to the previous decade. The population growth under age six in Karnataka registered negative with 8.2 per cent. If we look at the growth rates by districts it has been observed that, except Bangalore (10.5%), Gulbarga (2.6%) and Belgaum (2.4%), the rest of the districts had negative growth rate of child population. Further It was higher in Dharwad (–177%), Bijapur (–91%), Chitradurga (–80.5%), Raichur (–67%) Dakshin Kannada (–65.2%), Mysore (–50.3%) and Shimoga (–41.4%). The negative growth of child population in remaining districts was relatively lower.

If we look at the percentage change of male child population growth between two decades of 1981–1991 and 1991–2001, we observe that the district of Bangalore Urban has registered higher rate of growth with 33.35 per cent (Table 7.6). Also the districts of Kodagu and Chickmagalur have also had a positive growth with 4.51 and 1.52 per cent respectively. The growth rate change in the remaining districts in Karnataka was shown negative. Further it was reported that the maximum rate of growth in district of Dharwad (–185.45%), followed by Bijapur (–107.37%), Raichur (–92.50%), Chitradurga (–89%), Dakshin Kannada (–62%), Mysore (–54.79%) and Shimoga (–41.10%). Also refer Table 7.7 for the growth rate levels of male child population under age six in Karnataka by districts.

Growth Rate Trends and Levels: Female Child Population

In the previous part, we briefly explained the trends and levels of male child population in Karnataka. Now, we turn our attention towards the female child population growth and discuss the trends and levels by districts in Karnataka for the last two decades. It is clear from Table 7.8 that in the decade 1981–1991, female child population growth rate was about 5.7 per cent; but there was a drastic decline to 0.2 per cent by the decade 1991–2001. The average percentage change in the growth rate of female child population in Karnataka between the decades 1981–1991 and 1991–2001 was minus 5.5 per cent.

There was no significance difference of male and female child population growth in the decade 1991–2001. If we compare the status of gender balance in respect of the growth of male and female child population under age six was seems

Table 7.6

Districtwise Male/Female Population Growth Under Age 0–6 in Karnataka

S.No.	District	Decadal growth rate and change					
		Male			Female		
		1981–91	1991–01	Per cent increase or decrease	1981–91	1991–01	Per cent increase or decrease
1	Bangalore (U)	–22.81	10.5	33.35	–27.2	9.9	37.1
2	Bangalore R		–14.8	–14.81			0.0
3	Bagalkot			0.00			0.0
4	Belgaum	13.75	2.4	–11.33	12.4	–1.1	–13.5
5	Bellary	19.95	–14.6	–34.54	19.6	–15.9	–35.4
6	Bidar	21.93	–4.9	–26.80	23.7	–7.2	–30.9
7	Bijapur	16.18	–91.2	–107.37	15.0	–96.8	–111.8
8	Chamarajnagar			0.00			0.0
9	Chickmagalur	–6.68	–5.2	1.52	–7.4	–7.2	0.2
10	Chitradurga	8.52	–80.5	–89.00	5.6	9.9	4.3
11	Davanagere			0.00			0.0
12	Dharwad	8.34	–177.1	–185.45	8.5	–179.7	–188.2

Cont'd...

Cont'd...

13	Dakshin Kannada	–3.20	–65.2	–62.00	–4.2	–67.6	–63.5
14	Gadag			0.00			0.0
15	Gulbarga	21.53	2.6	–18.93	20.9	0.4	–20.5
16	Haveri			0.00			0.0
17	Hassan	–0.82	–18.8	–17.96	–4.7	–19.9	–15.3
18	Kolar	0.64	–5.2	–5.82	–2.1	–6.5	–4.4
19	Koppal			0.00			0.0
20	Kodagu	–7.01	–2.5	4.51	–3.4	–5.6	–2.2
21	Mandya	–6.59	–16.2	–9.58	–11.4	–19.2	–7.8
22	Mysore	4.52	–50.3	–54.79	4.0	–50.9	–54.9
23	Raichur	25.43	–67.1	–92.50	24.4	–67.1	–91.5
24	Shimoga	–0.20	–41.4	–41.15	–2.1	–42.1	–40.0
25	Tumkur	–3.08	–12.1	–9.06	–2.5	–14.6	–12.1
26	Udupi			0.00			0.0
27	Uttar Kannada	–1.22	–7.8	–6.62	–1.1	–8.2	–7.1
	Karnataka	**20.40**	**–8.2**	**–28.58**	**5.7**	**0.2**	**–5.5**

Note: Compiled from census data for the year 1981, 1991 and 2001 and growth rates calculated by the author.

Table 7.7

Growth Rate Levels of Male Child Population Under Age of 6 in Karnataka by Districts

Growth rates levels	*Districts (Decade 1981–1991)*	*1991–2001*
Negative (Growth Rates Less than 0)	Bangalore (U), Chickmagalur, Dakshin Kannada, Hassan, Kodagu, Mandya, Shimoga, Tumkur and Uttar Kannada	Dakshin Kannada and Dharwad
Very Low (Below 5%)	Kolar and Mysore	Bijapur and Raichur
Low (5.1–10)	Dharwad	Nil
Medium (10.1–15)	Belgaum	Nil
High (15.1–20)	Bellary and Bijapur	Chitradurga
Very High (20.1% or Greater)	Bidar, Chitradurga, Gulbarga and Raichur	Bangalore (U), Bangalore (R), Belgaum, Bellary, Bidar, Chickmagalur, Gulbarga, Hassan, Kolar, Kodagu, Mandya, Mysore, Shimoga, Tumkur and Uttar Kannada

Note: Classified by the author.

to be no any significance difference. By the statistical support one could note that in Karnataka female child population growth is slightly higher than male child population growth. It is evident from Table 5.6 that in decade 1991–2001 the male child population growth was absolutely negative, but on the other hand female child population growth was slightly positive with 0.2 per cent.

The percentage change between two decades in growth of female child population was highest in Dharwad (minus 188.2%), Bijapur (minus 111.8), Raichur (minus 91.5), Chitradurga (minus 88.6%), Dakshin Kannada (minus 63.4) and the southern district of Mysore (minus 54.9%). Excluding Bangalore (U) and Chickmagalur, all the districts registered below minus 50 per cent of change in the growth rate of female population. It ranged from minus 2.2 per cent in Kodagu to minus 35.5 per cent in Bellary.

Table 7.8 reveals that in decade the growth rate trend of female child population in decade 1981–1991 vary across districts. The growth rate of female child population was negative in most of the districts in southern region. But, it is quite the reverse in case of northern region. The districts of Bidar, Gulbarga, Bijapur, Belgaum and Raichur have shown high to very high growth rates level in female child population with 15–20 per cent or more. The districts of Dharwad and Chitradurga registered low (5.1–10%) rate of population growth. Interestingly the district of Mysore in southern region reported very low (below 5%) growth rate of female child population in the state.

There was a significant change in the growth rate of child population in decade 1991–2001, as compared with the previous decade of 1981–1991. As has already been mentioned, strong son preference, neglect of girl child due to increasing cost of marriage, education have influenced the negative growth of female child population not only in Karnataka, except Bangalore (U) and Gulbarga, but also in

India. It is observed from Table 5.8 that except the districts of Bangalore Urban and Gulbarga Chitradurga and Raichur and no other districts reported positive growth rate in female child population in Karnataka.

The positive growth rate of female child population in the above mentioned districts can be attributed to the two factors: (i) higher per cent of slum population in Bangalore, and (ii) low socio-economic status and, to some extent, religious sentiments in Gulbarga district. For example, the illiterates in the rural villages believe that a birth of child will be performed by God. Hence, they should not kill a born child irrespective of the gender. Probably certain extent these reasons and, to some extent, higher per cent of SCs/STs in Gulbarga were also influenced the positive growth of female child population.

Table 7.8

Decadal Growth of Female Child Population Under Age of 6 in Karnataka by District

Growth rate levels	***Districts (Decade 1981–1991)***	***1991–2001***
Negative (less than 0)	Bangalore (U), Chickmagalur, Dakshin Kannada, Hassan, Kolar, Kodagu, Mandya, Shimoga, Tumkur and Uttar Kannada	All districts excluding Gulbarga, Raichur, Chitradurga and Bangalore (U)
Very Low (below 5%)	Mysore	Gulbarga and Raichur
Low (5.1–10%)	Chitradurga and Dharwad	Bangalore (U)
Medium (10.1–15%)	Belgaum and Bijapur	Nil
High (15.1–20%)	Bellary	Chitradurga
Very High (20.1% or greater)	Bidar, Gulbarga and Raichur	Nil

Note: Classified by the author.

The reasons for positive growth of female child population in Bangalore Urban district can be seen in the context of highly polarized urban growth and consequent unusual concentration of population with unique demographic characteristics resulting in the creation of several slums in Bangalore metropolis. Further, it is to be noted that in poor families, the arrival of an additional child is considered as a source of income and a means of social security. Hence, poverty is closely associated with higher child population irrespective of the gender of child. These people (slum dwellers) do not think of their family welfare and improving their standard of living. Therefore, these factors led to higher fertility and also higher growth of child population. Lack of awareness about family planning, low standard of living and illiteracy etc., have influenced the birth of child. Hence, these aspects may be the reasons for positive growth in female child population in Bangalore Urban district. Of course, over the years, the governments and NGOs have taken some special initiative through planned programmes to improve the standard of slum dwellers. But there is a need to bring these people into the main stream. Still poverty and illiteracy are the drawbacks which continue to effect their lifestyle and livelihood.

8

Population Change among Scheduled Tribes in India

With Special Reference to Karnataka

As per notified schedule under Article 342 of the Constitution of India, there are 533 tribes concentrated across the states and union territories. India has the largest concentration of tribals, anywhere in the world except perhaps a certain country in Africa. Generally tribes are homogeneous in terms of socio-economic development unlike other groups. Majority of the Indian tribes are residing in remote areas, particularly hilly and forest regions. There are over 20 million tribals living below the poverty line. They live in the interior and fringes of forests. These tribes constitute the most backward groups of Indian society, and also each tribe is unique in terms of socio-cultural and economic organization. As per 2001 census, the total population of India was 1028.73 million. Of this, there were about 84.32 million of Scheduled Tribes (STs) contributing 8.8 per cent to the total population of India. The urban share of ST population in total population of STs in India as reported was that its proportion increased from 7.4 per cent in 1991 to 15.77 per cent in 2001.

Indian tribal studies, mostly done by anthropologists, have been remarkably largely closed to potentially useful influences from other disciplines such as economics and demography, resulting in the perditions, orientations and methodology adopted by the Indian anthropological discourse on tribes (Maharatna, 2005).

In this respect, the present study attempts to understand the rate of growth and its variation of ST population across states in India for the decades 1981–1991 and 1991–2001. The study has certain limitations and scope in analysing the population dynamics among STs in India. Over the years several studies have been carried out on tribal fertility and mortality by demographers and anthropologists who found similar findings about fertility and mortality trends of tribals in India. Hence the existing study did not focus on this issue. The study's aim is to understand the population dynamics which refers to total, rural and urban population of STs in India and its variation between the decades of 1981–1991 and 1991–2001.

In a historical perspective there has been some attention paid to study the demographic behaviour on Indian tribes which is available in the 19th and early 20th century (Davis, 1986; Bose, 1988; Singh, Premi, Bhatia, 1989; Ganagadharan, 1999; Maharatna, 2002). However, the study conducted by Gogoi (1990) observes that during 1961–1971 the rate of growth of tribal population in north-east India was lower than that of the general population. But, in case of Assam which was an exception it can be safely concluded that the migration of non-tribal population has taken place during the decade in the tribal dominated areas of the north-east. Another study conducted by Seikia in 1985, found that the natural increase of the tribal population in north-east region is very low during the decade 1971–1981. Further he pointed out that due to immigration into tribal areas of north-east region it has witnessed a higher growth rate of population.

The growth of Scheduled Tribe population in Karnataka was almost similar to that of general population until 1971. But due to inclusion of non-tribes into tribes there has been a phenomenal growth recorded in the decades of 1981–1991 and 1991–2001. Micro-level studies conducted jointly by the Government of India and United Nations in 1952 (UN, 1961), Karnataka Fertility Survey (1980) and Socio-Economic and Demographic Study on Soligas and Koragas have arrived at a conclusion that the increase in the proportion of children in the population is mostly due to the effects of rapid decline in child mortality even in the presence of fertility decline. A study conducted in 2000 by Mutharayappa on Kadukuruba and Jenukuruba who dominated tribes concentrated largely in H.D. Kote taluk in Mysore, the author arrives at conclusions that the contraceptive practices play a very important role in the fertility reduction of women in these particular groups.

The recent NFHS Surveys (1992–93 and 2003–04) records a tribal infant mortality rate as being lower than that of non-tribal lower caste people (SCs) by more than 18 per cent at the all-India level, and eight out of all Indian states show lower tribe infant mortality. There has always been a higher decadal rate of growth of the tribal population than that of the general population in the post-independence period. However, the gap in growth rates between the tribal and general population was highest during the 1951–61 and it seems to have narrowed down over the following decades (Maharatna, 2005).

There are several conceivable explanations for higher growth and concomitant rises in the tribal share in post-independence censuses. First, a substantial enlargement of the list of STs especially up to the late 1970s as well as the removal of area restrictions in 1976, certainly contributed to a relative swelling of the enumerated tribal population

(Beteille, 1986). Second, indeed fairly strong evidence suggests a higher real natural growth of the tribal population as compared to that of the total population. For instance, the decadal growth rate of the aggregate tribal population between 1961 and 1971, estimated on matched populations of Scheduled Tribes, turns out to be only about one per cent point lower (25.3%) than that (26.2%) based on unadjusted tribal populations in these censuses (Sinha, 1979). The available individual surveys of various tribes across Indian regions do not posit tribal fertility as always higher than that for non-tribal population groups (Nag, 1973).

India's relatively high tribal fertility refers to two facts, viz., (a) the tribals are primitive with presumably the reproductive behaviour of most aboriginal groups, and (b) their greater toleration of widow remarriage (Davis, 1951). The absence of child marriage practice among tribes in the past might have been a reason for tribal comparative mortality advantage in infancy, as the risk of death is generally higher among the infants of very young mothers. Understandably enough, a comparatively low tribal fertility itself (as a result longer duration of birth spacing as well as breast-feeding) could be a reason for a lower infant and child mortality (Agarwall, 1994).

Further, study by Wirsing 1985, indicated that especially prior to mass use of antibiotics and vaccinations that communities such as tribes who lived in less-crowded settlements and in great intimacy with the natural environment, generally fared better in mortality terms. Late marriage, gender relations and social organization to expect tribal fertility to have been lower than that of Hindus in the historical past (Randall, 1996). The out-migration of tribal population is relatively higher in advanced states of western and southern regions in the country since the mid-1970s. In fact, these factors were to a large extent true for the general population too, as is reflected in its slow down of growth rates although by a smaller magnitude (Maharatna, 2005).

Key Population and Literacy of Scheduled Tribes in India

The total population of India increased from 838.58 million in 1991 to 1028.73 million in 2001. Of the total, there were about 67.75 million of tribal population (1991) increased to 84.32 million in 2001. The proportion of Scheduled Tribe (ST) population in the total population of India was 8.08 and 8.19 per cent respectively for 1991 and 2001. It shows that, there was a slight increase of ST population in India from 8.08 per cent in 1991 to 8.19 per cent in 2001. But, it is quite reverse in the case of Scheduled Caste (SC) population, where the proportion slightly decreased. It can be seen in Table 8.1(a).

A decadal growth of total population in India was 23.85 per cent and 21.34 per cent for the respective decades of 1981–1991 and 1991–2001. The decadal growth rate of SCs and STs in India across states is presented in Table 8.1(b). In both the decades there was a higher growth rate of SCs and STs as compared to general population growth. However, it is noteworthy that in India due to continued effort by the Department of Health and Family Welfare in order to control population growth through certain policy interventions, it was observed that, in the decade 1991–2001 even the SC and ST population growth also declined along with the general population growth. But, still ST population growth has comparatively higher (19.64% 1991–2001) than the growth of SC population (17.5%) and also the general population growth (21.34%) in India for both the decades. This is due to various reasons which comprise demographic, social and economic aspects. Apart from this, the major reason for relative growth of STs in India was removal of area restriction following the 1976 Act. This section of the study presents more discussion on the issue.

It is evident that, the overall sex-ratio of general population in India has increased to 933 in 2001 from 927 in 1991 [Table 8.1 (b)]. However, it is important to note that the gender gap in sex-ratio was lower in ST population (969 females per 1,000 males) as compared to SC (916 females per 1,000 males) and also where the general population (927 per 1,000 males) is concerned. But, the progress of literacy among STs was lower than that of SC population in the country. In this view, it is quite relevant to understand the socio-economic status of ST and SC population to bring out the gaps. However, there have been studies which arrived at a conclusion that the tribal groups of Indian society are the most backward groups.

The ST population in the total population of India has shown that it was similar in 1991 and 2001. But, interestingly, it is noteworthy that the proportion of rural ST population in has declined considerably from 92.6 per cent in 1991 to 84.23 per cent in 2001. On the other hand the urban population of STs in India has increased obviously [Table 8.1 (a)].

Population Dynamics: Proportion Change

As per 2001 census, the percentage of ST population in the total population of India was highest in Madhya Pradesh (22.65%), Maharashtra (10.31%), Orissa (9.79%), Bihar (9.43%), Gujarat (8.99%), Rajasthan (8.53%), Andhra Pradesh (6.04%) and West Bengal (5.30%). Three-fourths of ST population, i.e., about 75 per cent exist in the above said states which also have come under top six states in India leading to higher percentage of ST population (Table 8.2). Remaining one-fourth (25%) of the ST population concentrated in the other states. The proportion was very low in union territories of Daman & Diu (0.02%), Andaman

Table 8.1(a)
Select Key Information on Population Aspects of India

Selected aspects	*Year*	
	1991	*2001*
Total general population	83,85,83,988	102,87,37,436
Total SC population	13,82,23,277	16,66,35,700
Total ST population	6,77,58,389	8,43,26,240
Percentage of SC population in the total general population	16.48	16.19
Percentage of ST population in the total general population	8.08	8.19
Percentage of male ST population in the total ST population	50.71	50.56
Percentage of female ST population in the total ST population	49.29	49.44
Percentage of rural ST population in the total ST population	92.6	84.23
Percentage of urban ST population in the total ST population	7.4	15.77

Source: Calculated by the author using census data.

Table 8.1(b)
Select Population Aspects of India

	Decadal growth rate		*Sex-ratio (7+)*		*Literacy*	
	1981–1991	*1991–2001*	*1991*	*2001*	*1991*	*2001*
Total	23.85	21.34	927	933	52.2	65.38
SC	24.21	17.5	916	936	37.4	54.69
ST	23.8	19.64	969	978	29.6	47.10

Source: Primary Census Abstract: Census of India 2001.

Nicobar Islands (0.04), Lakshdweep (0.07), Sikkim (0.13) and Dadra and Nagar Haveli (0.16%).

The proportion of ST population in the respective states of the total population: It is reported that the union territory of Lakshdweep, the states of Mizoram, Nagaland, Meghalaya, Arunachal Pradesh and the union territory of Dadra & Nagar Haveli, Manipur, Madhya Pradesh, Orissa, Gujarat, and Rajasthan which had the higher proportion of their total population. The percentage represented in these states in 2001 was 94.51 per cent, 94.45, 89.14, 85.94, 64.22, 62.23, 32.30, 23.21, 22.13, 14.76, and 12.56 per cent respectively. The percentage has been reported less than 10 per cent in the rest of the states with the state of Uttar Pradesh reporting the lowest (0.20%) and Bihar the highest (9.45%).

Percentage change across states between the years 1991 and 2001: It was reported that the percentage of ST population in the total population has slightly increased in the states of Bihar, Rajasthan, Andhra Pradesh, Karnataka, Meghalaya, Nagaland, Tripura, Tamil Nadu, Arunachal Pradesh, Kerala, Sikkim and Lakshadweep. Similarly, there has been slight decrease of its proportion in the total population in the rest of the states in the country.

Major Changes in the Growth Rate of ST Population

The average growth rate of ST population in India in the decade 1981–1991 was 24.85 per cent, it has declined to 18.58 per cent by the decade 1991–2001. In decade 1981–1991 the highest growth rate of Scheduled Tribe population in India was registered in Manipur (39.08%), Nagaland (39.42), Tripura (32.03), Meghalaya (29.84), Mizoram (29.68), Uttar Pradesh (28.19) and Dadra & Nagar Haveli (27.41%) with above national average rate of 24.85 per cent (Table 8.2). Only the states of Himachal Pradesh and Karnataka had registered low growth of ST population with

Table 8.2

Statewise Population Growth of STs in India

State/UTs	*Total population*		*%age in total India's population*		*%age in total state's population*		*Decadal growth rate*		*Decadal variation*
	1981	*1991*	*2001*	*[2001]*	*1991*	*2001*	*1981–91*	*1991–2001*	
1. M.P.	11867960	15399034	18850070	22.65	23.30	23.21	22.93	18.31	–4.62
2. Maharashtra	5645915	7318281	8577276	10.31	9.30	8.85	22.85	14.68	–8.17
3. Orissa	5834870	7032214	8145081	9.79	22.20	22.13	17.03	13.66	–3.36
4. Bihar	5732515	6616914	7845419	9.43	7.70	9.45	13.37	15.66	2.29
5. Gujarat	4788075	6161775	7481160	8.99	14.90	14.76	22.29	17.64	–4.66
6. Rajasthan	4130125	5474881	7097706	8.53	12.40	12.56	24.56	22.86	–1.70
7. A.P.	3119905	4199481	5024104	6.04	6.30	6.59	25.71	16.41	–9.29
8. W.B.	3036905	3808760	4406794	5.30	5.60	5.49	20.27	13.57	–6.69
9. Assam	CNC*	2874441	3308570	3.98	12.80	12.41	0.00	13.12	0.00
10. Karnataka	1803960	1915691	3463986	4.16	4.30	6.55	5.83	44.70	38.86
11. Meghalaya	1064965	1517927	1992862	2.39	85.50	85.94	29.84	23.83	–6.01
12. Nagaland	642661	1060822	1774026	2.13	87.70	89.14	39.42	40.20	0.78
13. Tripura	579976	853345	993426	1.19	30.90	31.05	32.03	14.10	–17.93
14. Mizoram	459597	653565	839310	1.01	94.70	94.45	29.68	22.13	–7.55

Cont'd...

Cont'd...

15. Manipur	385110	632173	741141	0.89	34.40	32.30	39.08	14.70	–24.38
16. Tamil Nadu	512555	574194	651321	0.78	1.00	1.04	10.73	11.84	1.11
17. Arunachal Pradesh	432775	550351	705158	0.85	63.70	64.22	21.36	21.95	0.59
18. Kerala	256220	320967	364189	0.44	1.10	1.14	20.17	11.87	–8.30
19. Uttar Pradesh	206740	287910	364092	0.44	0.20	0.20	28.19	20.92	–7.27
20. Himachal Pradesh	196968	218348	244587	0.29	4.20	4.02	9.79	10.73	0.94
21. D &N Haveli	79403	109380	137225	0.16	79.90	62.23	27.41	20.29	–7.11
22. Sikkim	73756	90901	111405	0.13	22.40	20.59	18.86	18.40	–0.46
23. Lakshadweep	37535	48163	57321	0.07	93.20	94.51	22.07	15.98	–6.09
24. A &N.Islands	22023	26770	29469	0.04	0.00	8.27	17.73	9.16	–8.57
25. Daman, Diu and Goa	10546	12100	14563	0.02	11.50	9.20	12.84	16.91	4.07
India Total	**50921060**	**67758389**	**83220261**	**100**	**8.80**	**8.19**	**24.85**	**18.58**	**–6.27**

Source: Census of India 1981,1991 and 2001Series 1, Part viii (b).

Note: *In state of Assam the census was not conducted in the year 1981. Total population excludes the states of Jammu & Kashmir, Punjab, Haryana and Pondicherry.

9.79 per cent and 5.83 per cent respectively. Though, the other states were registered below national average growth rate of 24.85 per cent.

If we look at the growth rate of ST population in the next decade of 1991–2001, there was a remarkable change in the growth rate of ST population (Table 8.2). The overall rate of growth of STs in the decade 1991–2001 has fallen down to 18.58 per cent as against 24.85 per cent in the preceding decade. The above said states like Nagaland, Manipur, Meghalaya, Mizoram, Uttar Pradesh, Dadra & Nagar Haveli had remained in the same position with higher rate of growth. It has an above national average of 18.58 per cent as compared to previous decade. Remaining all the states have registered a below state average rate of growth. Inclusion of new tribes in the schedule, a genuinely larger natural increase of the tribal population in the last two decades, the non-tribal population must have contributed to a rising tribal share in the total population in the post-independence period (Maharatna, 2005).

A remarkable higher growth rate of the tribal population during 1971–81 was due to inclusion of new tribes by removal of area restriction following the 1976 Act in the schedule, a genuinely larger natural increase of the tribal population in the last two decades, the non-tribal population must have contributed to a rising tribal share in the total population in the post-independence period. Tribal population is found in most parts of India, with a major proportion in the eastern, western and central regions, which together is home to nearly 90 per cent of the country's ST population. It is quite small both in northern and southern states. The share in the aggregate tribal population of the country was nearly doubled, over the period from 1961 to 1991 in the southern region (Maharatna, 2005). However, the increase in tribal share has not been uniform across individual states within the region. For instance, the increase has been negligible in Tamil

Nadu and even negative in Kerala (1991). But, southern states of Karnataka and Andhra Pradesh have experienced a big jump in their shares of tribal population; both within the state population as well as the country enumerated tribal population.

Enumeration biases relating to tribals which is perhaps relevant to a few states (particularly Karnataka and Maharashtra), the inter-state differentials in the growth of the tribal population should be shaped by regional variations in death and birth rates (i.e., natural growth of rates) and migration flows and patterns. In the case of a few tribal groups, the socio-political factors such as movement for inclusion of new tribal groups in the schedule. However, evidently anomalous situation has largely been created by the removal in 1976 of area restriction in identifying ST populations (Sinha, 1991). Here, one must note that Karnataka which has become a progressive state in southern India has registered higher (44.70%) rate of growth by increasing its proportion in the total population from 4.30 per cent in 1991 to 6.55 per cent in 2001. However, the substantial growth of ST population in Karnataka was not due to higher fertility nor influenced by the mortality ratio. It was mainly due to inclusion of new communities under the ST category, on removal of area restriction following the 1976 Act which has already been discussed earlier. The overall growth of general population in Karnataka has declined remarkably in the last two decades. Hence, here one could say that, the sustainable growth of this kind indicates the future growth of Karnataka in terms of socio-economic development.

Further, it may be noted that the growth rate of population among religion groups in Karnataka in the decade 1991–2001 was high among Muslims (23.48%), Christians (17.41%), Sikhs (51.72%), Buddhists (43.87%), and Jains (26.53%) as compared to Hindu growth rate of 15.32 per cent. In this view, we could state that the growth of population in Karnataka is not due to overall growth rates of population and Hindu religion in particular. It mainly concerns with the other religions of Muslim, Buddhist, and Jains and to some extent with Sikhs. Hence, the study suggest that there is need to give more attention towards the growth of these religion population groups to achieve sustainable development by using available natural resources within the region as well as in the state.

Hence, here one must note that presently Karnataka is recognized as a progressive state in India. But, in reality it seems that the state has failed to achieve development in individual aspects like reduction of poverty, providing employment for the youths and providing health care for the weaker sections of the society, equal growth of population among religion groups, creating awareness on family planning etc. Keeping this in mind the Government of Karnataka should now focus on these developmental issues especially with regard to weaker sections of the population, by providing employment and basic needs to the rural community.

There has been socio-economic disparity across the regions and the states in India. Of course, even if we look at the growth rate of population at national level, it has registered a steady decline, whereas at states and regional level it varies. Hence, we must give priority to the overall development of Karnataka rather than giving much attention to developed regions to bring people of all communities into the mainstream to achieve further goals for socio-economic development.

The reason behind the higher growth of ST population in states of Nagaland, Meghalaya, Mizoram, Arunachal Pradesh, Dadra and Nagar Haveli was that they had higher percentage (more than 75%) of STs in the total population of the respective states. However, the tribes of north-east are socio-economically better off than the other tribal groups in the mid-Indian region (Bhagat and Chattopadhyay, 2004). It is the higher percentage of its population in the total population of the states that has influenced the higher growth rate of ST population in these states. Further, one must note that the coefficient of the percentage of tribal population in total population of the respective states in India and the growth of tribal population has shown positive at 0.127, which means one per cent increase of tribal population in total population intends to increase 1.27 per cent of growth total in tribal population.

The most dominant groups in STs like Gond, Bhil, Munda and Santhal, the Bhil is the second largest tribe spread over large territory of western India. They are mainly concentrated in southern Rajasthan, Madhya Pradesh, Gujarat and northern Maharashtra. The study "Characteristics and Correlates of Tribal Fertility" conducted by Bhagat and Aparajita Chattopadhyay (2004), has revealed that among the four tribal groups the fertility rate show a higher in Bhils (3.6%) Gonds and Mundas (3.3%) than the other dominant tribe of Santhals (2.9%). Given this reason, probably it has influenced the higher growth of ST population in Rajasthan and Uttar Pradesh where the most dominant tribe, i.e., Gonds were concentrated. Uttar Pradesh has shown higher growth of tribal population in the decade 1991–2001.

The growth rate trend in the ST population between two decades was absolutely negative at the national level excepting the states of Karnataka (positive with higher growth of 38.86%), Daman & Diu (4.07%), backward state of Bihar (2.29%), Tamil Nadu (1.11%), Himachal Pradesh (0.94%), Nagaland (0.78), and Arunachal Pradesh (0.59%). These states should take special attention for reducing the ST population growth in India.

Dynamics of tribal population growth in India based on work participation rate, percentage of literacy rate and per cent of ST population in the total population of the respective states in India, the relationship between the growth of population and work participation of tribals represents the negative. The coefficient of work participation rate is very less significant (0.015) to influence the growth of population. The relationship between the literacy rate of tribal and growth of tribal population is positive at low level of significance, but the coefficient of literacy rate is negative, i.e., minus 1.041, representing the negative growth of population which also means that improvement in the literacy rate will have a negative impact on growth of population. The percentage of tribal population in total population of the respective state and growth of tribal population was positive at 0.127 which means one per cent increase in tribal population in total population intends to increase 1.27 per cent of growth in the total tribal population in India. The 't' value of per cent of ST population in total population of the state is significant at 5 per cent level.

Rural Population Growth and Variation

Table 8.3 describes that the average rural population growth of STs in India in decade 1981–1991 was 23.80%, it declined to 10.49 per cent in decade 1991–2001. The reduction of rural population growth rate between the decades was almost 13 per cent. If we examine the proportion of rural population by states in India it is observed that there are eight states, viz., Madhya Pradesh, Orissa, Maharashtra, Bihar, Gujarat, Rajasthan, Andhra Pradesh, and West Bengal which had the highest (75%) rural population in the country. Out of this Madhya Pradesh had three-fourths of proportion of ST population amongst eight states in India. The lower proportion of STs concentrated in the union territory of Daman & Diu (0.02%) and Assam (4.50%).

The decadal growth of rural population in India across states for the decade 1981–1991 and 1991–2001 has been reported in Table 8.3 and its explains that the north and north-eastern states of Manipur (41.19%), Nagaland (37.78%), Tripura (31.72%), Meghalaya (28.59%), Uttar Pradesh (928.18%), Dadra and Nagar Haveli, (27.48%), Sikkim (24.82%), Andhra Pradesh (24.59%) and Rajasthan (23.85%) registered higher growth rates and also dominated in rural population in the country. The states of Mizoram (1.54%), Lakshdweep (2.82%), and Karnataka (3.42%) had registered lower growth rates. The rural population growth rates in other states were between 10 and 20 per cent. The overall growth of rural population in decade 1991–2001 had declined to 10.49 per cent from 23.80 per cent from the previous decade of 1981–1991.

The rural population growth rates for the decade 1991–2001 of India when compared to the preceding decade, interestingly the progressive state of Karnataka was highest in the growth rate of rural population. The other few states also had higher growth rates which was above the national average rate of 10.49 per cent; they are Nagaland (39.56%), Lakshdweep (33.32%), Rajasthan (22.29%), Meghalaya (22.02%), with the rest of the states in the country between 10 to 20 per cent of growth in rural population. The union territory of Andaman and Nicobar Island and the southern state of Tamil Nadu registered a relatively low growth with below national average of 10.49 per cent.

The rural population growth in decade 1991–2001 has fallen in most of the states, except in few states which has been mentioned earlier. The reasons might be increasing infrastructure in cities and particularly metros like Kolkata, Chennai, Mumbai, Delhi, Hyderabad and Bangalore which have seen inclusive growth of urban population from rural areas. Especially, the youths and the male adults got employment in multi-national companies (MNCs) and other

Table 8.3

Statewise Rural Population Growth of STs in India

State/UTs	*Population*			*% age in total*	*Decadal growth rates*		*Decadal variation*
	1981	*1991*	*2001*		*1981–1991*	*1991–2001*	
Madhya Pradesh	11445965	14652730	17711283	25.26	21.89	17.27	–4.62
Orissa	5575330	6670506	7698358	10.98	16.42	13.35	-3.07
Maharashtra	5053195	6405814	7486537	10.68	21.12	14.44	-6.68
Bihar	5389830	6153659	7217716	10.30	12.41	14.74	2.33
Gujarat	4443165	5663178	6866637	9.79	21.54	17.53	–4.02
Rajasthan	3975325	5220549	6717830	9.58	23.85	22.29	-1.56
Andhra Pradesh	2926190	3880254	4646923	6.63	24.59	16.50	-8.09
West Bengal	2930120	3612448	4136366	5.90	18.89	12.67	-6.22
Assam	CNC*	2777308	3154546	4.50	0.00	11.96	11.96
Karnataka	1573840	1629496	2934530	4.19	3.42	44.47	41.06
Meghalaya	937013	1312093	1682670	2.40	28.59	22.02	-6.56
Nagaland	580601	933145	1544022	2.20	37.78	39.56	1.78
Tripura	573051	839264	967997	1.38	31.72	13.30	–18.42

Cont'd...

Cont'd...

Manipur	340484	578930	705912	1.01	41.19	17.99	–23.20
Arunachal Pradesh	424071	518222	606278	0.86	18.17	14.52	–3.64
Tamil Nadu	463365	505208	551143	0.79	8.28	8.33	0.05
Mizoram	352588	358113	430883	0.61	1.54	16.89	15.35
Kerala	251195	309764	350019	0.50	18.91	11.50	–7.41
Uttar Pradesh	194655	271035	336037	0.48	28.18	19.34	–8.84
Himachal Pradesh	193598	212940	237060	0.34	9.08	10.17	1.09
Dadra & Nagar Haveli	76776	105864	127410	0.18	27.48	16.91	–10.57
Sikkim	62762	83486	101909	0.15	24.82	18.08	–6.75
Andaman and Nicobar Islands	21854	26268	28456	0.04	16.80	7.69	–9.11
Lakshadweep	20873	21478	32209	0.05	2.82	33.32	30.50
Daman & Diu & Goa	8140	9281	11378	0.02	12.29	18.43	6.14
India Total	**47813986**	**62751033**	**70104109**	**100**	**23.80**	**10.49**	**–13.31**

Source: Census of India 1981,1991 and 2001Series 1, Part viii (b)

Note: *In state of Assam the census was not conducted in the year 1981. Total population excludes the states of Jammu & Kashmir, Punjab, Haryana and Pondicherry.

private sectors. Hence, with this background we could state that more and more people from rural areas were merging into cities and towns in India. In this inclusive population even STs might have also migrated. These migrants may be the workers working with construction, mining, quarrying and manufacturing sectors.

On the other hand as already mentioned earlier, the availability of employment opportunities in cities (both private and public sectors) like Bangalore (now it is called Bengaluru), Delhi, Kolkata, Chennai and Mumbai has influenced the moderate growth of rural population of STs in India through migration. Whereas the southern state of Karnataka was observed with positive growth with 41.06 per cent of rural population both in the decades of 1981–1991 and 1991–2001. The reasons for higher growth have already been stated in the earlier discussion. Its growth ranks first in the country followed by Lakshdweep (+ 30.50%), Mizoram (+15.35%), Dadra and Nagar Haveli (+0.14%), Bihar (+0.33%), Himachal Pradesh (+0.09), and Tamil Nadu (+0.05%). In most of the states the decadal variation between 1981–1991 and 1991–2001 was absolutely negative.

Urban Population Growth and Variation

Under the impact of globalization and economic liberalization, studies on urbanization and migration have become important in the development aspect especially for developing countries like India. In this context we concentrate our interest on urban population of STs in India, and as per 2001 census, the state of Madhya Pradesh has the higher percentage (15.73%) of urban population of STs in India. This is followed by Maharashtra (15.73%), Bihar, (9.05%), Gujarat (8.86%), Karnataka (7.63%), Orissa (6.44%), Mizoram (5.89%), and Rajasthan (5.48%). These states constitute almost 81 per cent of total urban population of STs in the country (see Table 8.4). The bottom states and union territories in terms of low percentage of ST urban population were Daman & Diu, and Goa (0.05%), Andaman Nicobar Islands (0.01%), and rest of the states had shown very less percentage of urban population in the total population of India (Table 8.4). If we look at the urbanization through STs in India across states it can be observed that the urban population growth of Scheduled Tribes in India was 37.87 per cent in decade 1981–1991 which decreased to 27.81 per cent in decade 1991–2001. However, it indicates that the urban population growth has been registered above the national average of general population with 24.38 per cent.

In decade 1981–1991 among the states and union territories in India, Arunachal Pradesh, Mizoram, Tripura, Kerala, Nagaland, West Bengal, Madhya Pradesh, Andhra Pradesh, and Rajasthan have registered higher growth rate of urban population with above the national average of 37.87 per cent. Interestingly, the state of Sikkim had shown negative rate of growth and the rest of the states were under below national average rate of 37.87 per cent. In decade 1991–2001, few states like Karnataka, Uttar Pradesh, and Tamil Nadu were included in this group, i.e., above the national average rate of growth of 27.81 per cent. The north-eastern state of Arunachal Pradesh ranks first in the growth of urban population (67.51%) in India and it is followed by Dadra and Nagar Haveli (64.18%), Andaman Nicobar Islands (50.44%), Karnataka (45.95%), Tripura (44.63%), Nagaland (44.49%), Uttar Pradesh (39.85%), Meghalaya (33.64%), Rajasthan (33.05%), Tamil Nadu (31.14%) and Himachal Pradesh (28.14%). The state of Manipur and the union territory of Lakshdweep had registered negative rate of growth in urban population. The below national average rate of growth was concentrated in other states of India.

Table 8.4
Statewise Urban Population Growth of STs in India

State/UTs	*Population*			*%age in total*	*Decadal growth rates*		*Decadal variation*
	1981	*1991*	*2001*		*1981–1991*	*1991–2001*	
Maharashtra	592720	912467	1090739	15.73	35.04	16.34	–18.70
Madhya Pradesh	421995	746304	1138787	16.42	43.46	34.47	–8.99
Gujarat	344910	498597	614523	8.86	30.82	18.86	–11.96
Bihar	342685	463255	627703	9.05	26.03	26.20	0.17
Orissa	259540	361708	446723	6.44	28.25	19.03	–9.22
Andhra Pradesh	193715	319227	377181	5.44	39.32	15.37	–23.95
Mizoram	107009	295452	408427	5.89	63.78	27.66	–36.12
Karnataka	230120	286195	529456	7.63	19.59	45.95	26.35
Rajasthan	154800	254332	379876	5.48	39.13	33.05	–6.09
Meghalaya	127952	205834	310192	4.47	37.84	33.64	–4.19
West Bengal	106785	196312	270428	3.90	45.60	27.41	–18.20
Nagaland	62060	127677	230004	3.32	51.39	44.49	–6.90
Assam	CNC*	97133	154024	2.22	0.00	36.94	36.94
Tamil Nadu	49190	68986	100178	1.44	28.70	31.14	2.44

Cont'd...

Cont'd...

Manipur	44626	53243	35229	0.51	16.18	–51.13	–67.32
Arunachal Pradesh	8704	32129	98880	1.43	72.91	67.51	–5.40
Lakshdweep	20873	26685	25112	0.36	21.78	–6.26	–28.04
Uttar Pradesh	12085	16875	28055	0.40	28.39	39.85	11.47
Tripura	6925	14081	25429	0.37	50.82	44.63	–6.19
Kerala	5025	11203	14170	0.20	55.15	20.94	–34.21
Sikkim	10994	7415	9496	0.14	–48.27	21.91	70.18
Himachal Pradesh	3370	5409	7527	0.11	37.70	28.14	–9.56
Dadra & Nagar Haveli	2627	3516	9815	0.14	25.28	64.18	38.89
Daman & Diu and Goa	2406	2819	3185	0.05	14.65	11.49	–3.16
Andaman & Nicobar Islands	169	502	1013	0.01	66.33	50.44	–15.89
India Total	**3111285**	**5007356**	**6936152**	**100**	**37.87**	**27.81**	**–10.06**

Source: Census of India 1981,1991 and 2001Series 1, Part viii (b)

Note: *In state of Assam the census was not conducted in the year 1981. Total population excludes the states of Jammu & Kashmir, Punjab, Haryana and Pondicherry.

The variation in the growth of ST population in India between two decades of 1981–1991 and 1991–2001 was highest in Sikkim (70.8%). This is followed by union territory of Dadra and Nagar Haveli (38.89%), Karnataka (26.35%), Uttar Pradesh (11.47%), Tamil Nadu (2.44%), and Bihar (0.17%).

Male/Female Population Growth and Variation

The average decadal growth of tribal male population was 25.47 per cent in the decade 1981–1991; it was came down to 17.79 per cent in decade 1991–2001. Generally, there was fall in the growth rates of STs during the decade between 1981–1991 and 1991–2001. The northern state of Manipur registered higher growth of ST males in decade 1981–1991. Interestingly, the state of Karnataka has the lowest growth with 6.64 per cent of ST male population in the country. Most of the northern states like Meghalaya, Nagaland, Tripura, Mizoram, and Uttar Pradesh, Dadra & Nagar Haveli had the growth rates above national average of 25.47 per cent. The growth rates in other states had shown below national average and also relatively moderate growth of male population (Table 8.5).

In decade 1991–2001 there was a sudden jump in the growth of ST male in Karnataka which has registered a phenomenal growth with 44.38 per cent. In the earlier decade it conversely registered low growth rate with merely 6.64 per cent and which was the lowest in the country. There was a remarkable decline of ST male population growth in Nagaland, Tripura and Manipur. The decadal variation was minus 26 per cent for Manipur, minus 18.22 per cent in Tripura and minus 13.06 per cent in Nagaland. This is due to male migration to other states like Karnataka, Maharashtra and also to the metro cities in other parts of India. On the other hand southern state of Karnataka and the state of

Assam had shown positive growth with a decadal variation of 37.74 per cent and 12.90 per cent respectively. Even the of Daman & Diu (1.85%), Bihar (0.50%) and Himachal Pradesh (0.03%) had shown positive growth with low percentage. The decadal variation in rest of the states registered from minus 2.43 per cent (Sikkim) to minus 10.56 per cent (Andhra Pradesh), i.e., 39.79 per cent in decade 1981–1991 to 13.78 per cent in decade 1991–2001.

Table 8.6 presents the decadal growth of female population for the decades 1981–1991 and 1991–2001. The average decadal growth of female population in decade 1981–1991 was 24.07 per cent. Among the states Nagaland and Manipur had highest rate of growth with 38.86 and 38.34 per cent respectively. Even the states of Tripura (31.95%), Meghalaya (929.87%), Mizoram (29.09%) Uttar Pradesh (28.96%), Dadra and Nagar Haveli (25.28%), Andhra Pradesh (24.92%), Rajasthan (23.61%), Madhya Pradesh (22.18%), Maharashtra (21.97%), Gujarat (21.55%) and Union Territory of Lakshadweep had highest rate of ST female population growth in decade 1981–1991. The rate of growth in rest of the states was below 20 per cent and further the lowest rate of growth was observed in the states of Karnataka (4.99%), Himachal Pradesh (9.57%) and Bihar (12%).

In the decade 1991–2001, the national average rate of female population growth had absolutely declined from 24.07 per cent in decade 1981–1991 to 18.86 per cent in decade 1991–2001. Excepting the states of Karnataka, Bihar, Nagaland, Tamil Nadu, Arunachal Pradesh, Himachal Pradesh, Sikkim and Daman & Diu there were no states that registered increasing growth of female population in the decade 1991–2001 as compared to previous decade. The reasons are similar which have already been cited in the earlier part.

Table 8.5

Statewise Male Population Growth of STs in India

State/UTs	Population			Decadal growth rates		Decadal variation
	1981	1991	2001	1981–91	1991–2001	
Madhya Pradesh	5921795	7758174	9482574	23.67	18.18	–5.49
Orissa	2887485	3512891	4066783	17.80	13.62	–4.18
Bihar	2864190	3357563	3959074	14.69	15.19	0.50
Maharashtra	2836525	3717783	4347754	23.70	14.49	–9.21
Gujarat	2411265	3131947	3790117	23.01	17.37	–5.65
Rajasthan	2115075	2837014	3650982	25.45	22.29	–3.15
Andhra Pradesh	1575660	2142817	2548295	26.47	15.91	–10.56
West Bengal	1537500	1938955	2223924	20.70	12.81	–7.89
Assam	CNC*	1461560	1678117	0.00	12.90	12.90
Karnataka	911885	976744	1756238	6.64	44.38	37.74
Meghalaya	533569	760234	996567	29.82	23.71	–6.10
Nagaland	533569	760234	913203	29.82	16.75	–13.06
Tripura	294778	434225	504320	32.11	13.90	–18.22

Cont'd...

Cont'd...

Tamil Nadu	260460	293012	328917	11.11	10.92	–0.19
Mizoram	230022	329819	422963	30.26	22.02	–8.24
Arunachal Pradesh	213550	275397	352017	22.46	21.77	–0.69
Manipur	194313	322720	374319	39.79	13.78	–26.00
Kerala	128095	160812	180169	20.34	10.74	–9.60
Uttar Pradesh	109070	150429	187168	27.49	19.63	–7.87
Himachal Pradesh	99201	110240	122549	10.01	10.04	0.03
Dadra and Nagar Haveli	38757	54102	67663	28.36	20.04	–8.32
Sikkim	38479	47504	56940	19.00	16.57	–2.43
Lakshadweep	18663	24160	28611	22.75	15.56	–7.20
Daman & Diu &Goa	5369	6272	7489	14.40	16.25	1.85
Andaman Nicobar Islands	11286	13750	15127	17.92	9.10	–8.82
India Total	**25770561**	**34578358**	**42061880**	**25.47**	**17.79**	**–7.68**

Source: Census of India 1981,1991 and 2001Series 1, part viii (b)
Note: *In state of Assam the census was not conducted in the year 1981. Total population excludes the states of Jammu & Kashmir, Punjab, Haryana and Pondicherry

Table 8.6

Statewise Female Population Growth of STs in India

State/UTs	*Female population*			*Decadal growth rate*		*Decadal variation*
	1981	*1991*	*2001*	*1981–1991*	*1991–2001*	
Madhya Pradesh	5946165	7640860	9367496	22.18	18.43	–3.75
Orissa	2947385	3519323	4078298	16.25	13.71	–2.55
Bihar	2868325	3259351	3886345	12.00	16.13	4.14
Maharashtra	2809390	3600498	4229522	21.97	14.87	–7.10
Gujarat	2376810	3029828	3691043	21.55	17.91	–3.64
Rajasthan	2015050	2637867	3446724	23.61	23.47	–0.14
Andhra Pradesh	1544245	2056664	2475809	24.92	16.93	–7.99
West Bengal	1499405	1869805	2182870	19.81	14.34	–5.47
Assam	CNC*	1412881	1630453	0.00	13.34	13.34
Karnataka	892075	938947	1707748	4.99	45.02	40.03
Meghalaya	531396	757693	996295	29.87	23.95	–5.92
Nagaland	315292	515666	860823	38.86	40.10	1.24
Tripura	285198	419120	489106	31.95	14.31	–17.64

Cont'd...

Cont'd...

Tamil Nadu	252095	281182	322404	10.34	12.79	2.44
Mizoram	229575	323746	416347	29.09	22.24	–6.85
Arunachal Pradesh	219225	274954	353141	20.27	22.14	1.87
Manipur	190797	309453	366822	38.34	15.64	–22.70
Kerala	128125	160155	184020	20.00	12.97	–7.03
Uttar Pradesh	97670	137481	176924	28.96	22.29	–6.66
Himachal Pradesh	97767	108109	122038	9.57	11.41	1.85
Dadra and Nagar Haveli	40646	55278	69562	26.47	20.53	–5.94
Sikkim	35277	43397	54465	18.71	20.32	1.61
Lakshadweep	18872	24003	28710	21.38	16.39	–4.98
Daman & Diu and Goa	5177	5828	7074	11.17	17.61	6.44
Andaman Nicobar Islands	10737	13020	14342	17.53	9.22	–8.32
India Total	**25356699**	**33395109**	**41158381**	**24.07**	**18.86**	**–5.21**

Source: Census of India 1981,1991 and 2001Series 1, Part viii (b).

Note: *In state of Assam the census was not conducted in the year 1981. Total population excludes the states of Jammu & Kashmir, Punjab, Haryana and Pondicherry.

When we analyse the decadal variation between the two decades of 1981–1991 and 1991–2001, it was observed that the national average growth rate between these decades was minus 5.21 per cent. There was a negative rate of ST females' population growth in most of the states, excepting Karnataka, Bihar, Nagaland, Arunachal Pradesh and Daman & Diu. Probably this is due to migration.

9

Health Care Infrastructure in Karnataka

The key objective of the Ministry of Health and Family Welfare is to provide basic health care services to the people of India. Indeed, the health care programmes have greatly improved the situation in delivering the health care services over the years. Over 50 years, India has seen visible achievements in health care services as well as improvements in health care facilities especially in primary health care, both in rural and urban sectors. The motto "Health for All" by the World Health Organization (WHO) is visible today. Nevertheless, in India there are still major weaknesses in health care administration as well as in the organization which have been aggravated by population pressure and financial limitations.

However, the most important shortcomings relate not only to the regional coverage of health care but also quality of primary health care in respect of poor and vulnerable groups. The problems are rooted in over-centralized management structure, cumbersome administrative procedures and weak participation of regional authorities and local communities. Of course, over the years, the health status of the people of India has improved, but it has to reach its further goal. However, in certain pockets, malnutrition and unsanitary health environment happen to be the main causes for widespread diseases such as gastro-enteritis, respiratory infections, malaria and tuberculosis. Although, the mortality rate has come down in the recent years on the other hand morbidity is increasing.

In India, after independence, there has been a great expansion of health services in the decentralized health care reforms through Primary Health Centres (PHCs), Community Health Centres (CHCs) and also Sub-Centres (SCs). However, the functioning of the health care system at secondary and tertiary level is not up to desired expectations. Even the 10th Plan (1997–2000) has admitted it and cited a number of factors responsible for inefficient functioning.

To provide and facilitate health care services in India, the Union Government appointed a committee in 1943 under the chairmanship of Sir Joseph Bhore (popularly known as Bhore Committee) submitted its report in 1946. The Government accepted its recommendations and implemented the same for effective services in the health care sector. Keeping in view, the recommendations of the committee, sub-centres and primary health centres were set up in the rural areas in the ratio of one for 20,000 population and one for 100,000 population respectively with a view to providing health care services to the people.

Thereafter, over a period of time, the population served by these centres were reduced. Subsequently, other committees were set up by the Government of India, among which the important ones were the Mudaliar Committee in 1961, Srinivasan Committee in 1970, the Mukherji Committee in 1974 and further the National Health Policies of the Government of India were formulated in 1983 and 2002.

As a result of all these efforts, today primary health care is accessible to all people including the rural and weaker sections of the society. However, increasing number of private health institutions have been providing a good health services in the country but, these institutions were mostly established in the urban areas, and hence, only the rich and to certain extent the middle class people can access these expensive health care facilities.

In this context, this chapter presents the overall health care infrastructure in Karnataka with the available data called out from the Department of Health and Family Welfare, Government of Karnataka. The emphasis of the public health care system has been on meeting the basic health care needs of the poorer sections of the population on a free or subsidized basis. After almost 50 years of such an expansion and diversification of health care services in the country, now one can assess how the public health care services including the curative services are reaching the people and how this expansion has benefitted to the people of India.

The general impression emerging from various studies (which are widely quoted in India and abroad) indicates that the public health care system which include the network of PHCs and CHCs and also district hospitals does not serve the needs of the poor whom they are intended to serve. Here, I have tried to address the various aspects of health amenities; which include average area, rural population as well as number of villages covered by each Primary Health Centre, Community Health Centre, and Sub-Centre. In addition we have presented an analysis of population and doctor ratio, ANM population ratio and nurse-bed ratio etc. An analysis has been done on the manpower in the health system in Karnataka.

Health Amenities

In the post-independence period, the health care infrastructure both at the national and state level has enhanced and improved. Presently, Karnataka has 177 public hospitals, 301 CHCs, 1,679 PHCs, 578 PHUs and 8,143 Sub-Centres which serving the health care sector. Interestingly, total number of private medical colleges are higher than public medical colleges in the state, i.e., 28 and 4 respectively. There are 269 rural and 87 urban family welfare centres including 4 health and family welfare training centres working in Karnataka. For every 637 sq km there is one CHC and similarly for every 114 sq km there is one PHC. And each sub-centre serves about 23 sq km of area in the state (Table 9.1).

If we look at the population served by each CHC, PHC and SC in the year 2005–2006 in Karnataka it becomes clear that each CHC served about 1,15,910 rural population, and each PHC served about 20,780 rural population and each SC served about 4,284 rural population in the state. On the other hand average number of villages covered by each CHC, PHC and SC were 92, 16 and 3 respectively.

Further, there was one government doctor for every 10,385 people. And doctor patient ratio was 1: 6,346 and for every 3,896 population there was one ANM working in the health care sector in Karnataka.

In the year 2004–05 there were 3,76,960 people who underwent sterilization accounting to 91 per cent in the target. The IUD insertions were about 2,98,625 accounting 92.5 per cent in the target. Similarly immunization programme covered about 10,77,554 BCG, 10,61,788 DPT, measles 10,04,958 and TT injection for pregnant women were 11,18,524.

In Karnataka, there are a total 5,065 sanctioned posts of doctors. Out of which about 4,414 posts have been filled and rest of the posts have fallen vacant. About 229 dental doctors are working and no vacant position exists in this category.

However, many staff nurse posts are vacant. As per the year 2004–05 there were 4,479 ANMs working in the total sanctioned posts of 4,717. About 875 senior male health assistant working as against the total sanctioned posts of 1,302. Similarly, there are 4,022 junior male health assistants working as against the total sanctioned posts of 5,853. Coming to the senior female health assistants there are 1,067 out of 1,219 sanctioned posts. The working strength of junior female health assistants in the public health department were 9,376 out of 10,255 sanctioned posts.

Table 9.1

Health Amenities and Manpower in Karnataka (2005–06)

No. of Hospitals	177
No. of PHCs	1679
No. of Community Health Centres	253
No. of PHUs	581
No. of Sub-Centres	8143
No. of Urban PHCs	17
No. of Maternity Annex	304
No. of Beds	43158
No. of Government Medical Colleges	4
Central Government Hospitals and Dispensaries	26
ESI Hospitals and Dispensaries	136
Local Body Hospitals and Dispensaries	53
Rural Family Welfare Centres	269
Urban Family Welfare Centres	87
Urban Health Centres	124
Post Partum Centres	103
Medical Termination of Pregnancy (MTP) Centres	517
Health Family Welfare Training Centres	4

Cont'd...

.Cont'd...

Rural Population Covered by each Sub-Centre	4275
Rural Population Covered by a each PHC	20760
Average area covered (sq km) by each Sub-Centre	23.55
Average area covered (sq km) by each PHC	114.36
Average area covered (sq km) by each CHC	770.24
Average No. of Villages covered by each Sub-Centre	3
Average No. of Villages covered by each PHC	16
Average No. of Villages covered by each CHC	109
Government Doctor: Population Ratio	1:10260
Doctor: Population ratio including Teaching Staff	1:3240
Doctor: Patient Ratio	1:2167
ANM: Population Ratio	1:4275
Nurse: Bed Ratio	1:9

Health Manpower

Category	*Sanctioned*	*Working*
Doctors	5089	4496
Dental Doctors	246	173
Staff Nurse	5317	4309
Senior Health Assistant (M)	1302	875
Junior Health Assistant (M)	5853	2873
Senior Health Assistant (F)	1219	1067
Junior Health Assistant (F)	10255	8955
Laboratory Technicians	2519	858
Pharmacists	2661	1243
X-Ray Technicians	327	227
Refractionists	515	385

Source: Karnataka Health Profile, 2005–2006, Directorate of Health & Family Welfare Services, Bangalore.

There is a huge shortage of junior male health assistants in Karnataka. There are 2,980 junior health assistant posts vacant. Similarly, there were 1,300 junior female health assistant posts are vacant. A major problem in the rural health care is that there is shortage of doctors. As already noted that, out of 5,089 vacancies of doctors about 593 posts are vacant (2004–05). In this background one can draw a conclusion that the problem of rural health care system and also its functioning system in Karnataka is not extremely good and hence, it needs to be strengthened. No doubt, Karnataka has achieved certain goals in the primary health care, but, it has to strive further so as to provide health care facilities for their rural poor and the vulnerable groups.

Children's Health Care Infrastructure in Karnataka

In order to understand health care Infrastructure for children in Karnataka, an effort has been made in this chapter to analyse the collected information from the primary source on health aspects of child population by districts. Data relating to working status of the doctors, existing health care facilities, Children's Out-Patient Department (COPD) etc., has been briefly discussed. Further, an attempt has been done to report the exiting health care services for children by analysing health care infrastructure like using modern equipments like ultrasound, laser, fiber optic endoscopy and microscope. The detailed analysis has been done to report the public health care facilities provided by COPD, in district hospitals in Karnataka during the study period February to March 2006. Here also, emphasis has been given to understand the special services like neo-natal incentive care unit (NICU) and baby clinic for health care of children in Karnataka.

Working Status of Doctors

The working status of doctors in children's OPDs in district hospitals, number of sanctioned posts, working doctors, vacant posts etc., has been reported in this section. During the study period, it was reported that the total number of sanctioned posts of children's doctors in district hospitals of Karnataka stood at 53 – the districts of Belgaum, Gulbarga and Kolar having three posts each, followed by districts like Bellary, Chickmagalur, Chitradurga, Hassan and Uttar Kannada and Tumkur with two posts each. The rest of the districts (Bidar, Chamarajnagar, Dharwad, Gadag, Kodagu Raichur, Shimoga and Udupi) had one doctor each.

Regarding the working status of doctors in district hospitals during the study period, it was reported that there were no permanent doctors at children's OPDs in newly constituted districts like Bagalkot, Haveri, Koppal and Bijapur. During that time temporary doctors were found attending the cases in these COPDs (Table 9.2).

In the districts of Tumkur, Kolar, Davanagere, Gulbarga and Shimoga the out-surgeons (trainee doctors) had been found attending on the patients in COPD. Here it was reported that the out-surgeons must do the training in general hospitals for a period of one year after completion of their two years course of MBBS. As a result, these districts benefitted from their service. However, it was observed from the field information that in COPD the regular doctors had given all the responsibilities to the out-surgeons for health check-up. Further, we found doctors working on a contract basis in children's OPD, in district hospitals like Belgaum, Davanagere, Dakshin Kannada, Gulbarga and Mysore.

The vacant posts of children doctors in district hospitals of Karnataka were 16 out of 53. During the study period there were no permanent children's doctors in district hospitals of Bagalkot, Haveri, and Koppal. Temporary doctors were found attending the cases at children's OPD during the time of visit. However, here one could note that they were newly carved districts in 2004. Of course, there is a

Table 9.2
Working Status of Doctors in Children Out-Patient Department (COPD) in District Hospitals in Karnataka (2006–2007)

District	*No. of sanctioned posts*	*No. of working doctors*	*No of vacant posts*
Bagalkot	2	Nil	2
Bellary	2	2	Nil
Belgaum	3	2+3*	Nil
Bidar	2	1	1
Bijapur	2	Nil	2
Chamarajnagar	2	1	1
Chickmagalur	2	2	Nil
Chitradurga	2	2	Nil
Davanagere	2	2+1	Nil
Dharwad	2	1	1
Dakshin Kannada	2	2+1	Nil
Gadag	2	1	Nil
Gulbarga	3	3+3	Nil
Haveri	2	Nil	2
Hassn	2	2	Nil
Kolar	3	3	Nil
Koppal	2	Nil	2
Kodagu	2	1	1
Mandya	2	2	Nil
Mysore	2	2+1	Nil
Raichur	2	1	1
Shimoga	2	1	1
Tumkur	2	1	1
Udupi	2	1	1
Uttar Kannada	2	2	Nil
Karnataka	**53**	**44**	**16**

Source: Field survey during February-March, 2006.
Note: *Working on contract basis.

need to appoint permanent doctors for these hospitals immediately. There are also vacant posts of children's doctors in district hospitals of Bidar, Chamarajnagar, Dharwad, Kodagu, Raichur, Shimoga and Udupi. But, it was found that there were no vacant posts in most of the southern districts and the districts of Bellary, Belgaum, Gadag, Gulbarga which come under the northern region.

A common response by the hospital authorities for not filling the vacant posts of children's doctors in district hospitals in Bidar, Chamarajnagar, Dharwad, Gadag, Kodagu, Shimoga and Udupi was that the government had not filled them. During our survey period a permanent doctor working in COPD in district hospital in Raichur took voluntary retirement.

Available Health Care Facilities for Children in Karnataka

To review the existing health care infrastructure facilities in children's OPD in district hospitals, information relating to children's ward, bed strength and also neo-natal incentive care unit (NICU) and its special care has been collected. In this regard Table 9.3 presents the status of children's ward in district hospitals of Karnataka excluding Bangalore and Bangalore Urban. The district hospitals of Gulbarga, Bidar and Kolar had three children's ward in their general hospitals. Rest of the districts had either one or two wards in their hospitals. This can be observed from Table 9.3. There was special information by the district hospitals of Raichur that there was a special ward called GE (gastro enteritis) ward. It is only meant for diarrhoea patients. This was reported at the district hospital of Raichur, and no other district hospital had this facility.

If we look at the bed strength in children's ward by district hospitals, the higher number of beds were found in the children wards in the district hospitals of Gulbarga (90), Davanagere (80), Mysore and Dakshin Kannada (60). Lower number of beds for children was found in the district of Bijapur (10), Raichur (12), and Mandya (22). Remaining district hospitals had 30 to 40 beds in their children wards. Here it was reported that there was a special ward, called neo-natal incentive care unit (NICU) existing in many district hospitals in Karnataka. This facility is mainly meant for new born babies who weighted below 1.5 kg.

The available information on this aspect has been cited in Table 9.3. It was reported that this facility did not exist in district hospitals of Bagalkot, Bidar, Bijapur, Chamarajnagar, Gadag, Haveri, Kolar, Koppal and Udupi. The rest of the districts reported of NICU facility in their hospitals.

As per the collected information on NICU and its bed strength the bed strength at NICU ranged from 4 to 20. Comparatively the districts of Gulbarga, Tumkur (4) and Raichur (5) had fewer numbers of beds in their NICU (Table 9.3). The number of bed strength in the NICU in other districts ranged from 10 to 20.

Status of Out-Patients and In-Patients in District Hospitals

To know the existing status of children's OPD, we tried to understand the information collected on the status of out-patients coming for health check-up, and in-patients on a routine basis. In this regard Table 9.4 presents an average number of patients coming for health check-up, and average number of patients getting admitted for further treatment as in-patients in COPD in district hospitals.

According to our survey an average of 200–230 patients come for health check-up in Bidar, and this is the highest in Karnataka. Second highest number of patients came for health check-up in Kolar and Tumkur (180–200). In districts

Table 9.3
Available Health Facilities in District Hospitals for Children in Karnataka

District	*No. of children's ward*	*No. of beds*	*NICU***	*No. of beds*
Bagalkot	1	30	N	—
Bellary	2	40	Y	20
Belgaum	1	40	Y	10
Bidar	3	30	N	—
Bijapur	1	10	N	—
Chamarajnagar	1	30	N	—
Chickmagalur	1	30	Y	10
Chitradurga	1	40	Y	10
Davanagere	2	80	Y	20
Dharwad	1	40	Y	10
Dakshin Kannada	2	60	Y	10
Gadag	1	30	N	—
Gulbarga	2	90	Y	4
Haveri	1	30	N	—
Hassan	1	30	Y	10
Kolar	3	30	N	—
Koppal	1	30	N	—
Kodagu	1	30	Y	10
Mandya	2	22	Y	10
Mysore	2	60	Y	20
Raichur	1+1*	12	Y	5
Shimoga	1	30	Y	18
Tumkur	1	60	Y	20
Udupi	1	40	N	—
Uttar Kannada	1	30	Y	10

Source: Field survey during February-March, 2006.
Note: *GE ward (gastro enteritis) ** Neo-natal incentive care unit. Y indicates Yes, and N indicates No.

like Raichur and Davanagere, an average number of patients coming for health check-up ranged from 100–120 per day. In the districts of Bellary, Chitradurga, Hassan, Mysore and Udupi, the number varied from 80–100. In the rest of the districts like Bijapur, Chickmagalur, Dharwad, Gadag, Koppal, Kodagu, Mandya and Shimoga the number ranged from 60–80 per day. Comparatively less number of children patients came to hospitals for health check in Uttar Kannada and Belgaum (50–60). There were 30–40 patients coming for health check-up per day in Haveri district.

Further, we have focused on the number of people coming to hospitals both as out-patients and in-patients in COPD. In Table 9.4, column 4 provides information on the number of cases admitted for further health care in the hospitals. It is reported there were 8–12 patients admitted for further health care in hospitals of Kolar, Bidar, Davanagere and Raichur, followed by Bagalkot, Belgaum, Chitradurga, Dakshin Kannada Gadag, Gulbarga, Mandya and Mysore (4–8). Relatively less (4–8) number of patients were admitted for further health treatment in districts of Bellary, Chamarajnagar, Chickmagalur, Dharwad, Haveri, Koppal, Kodagu, Shimoga, Udupi, Uttar Kannada and Tumkur.

Very less number of patients admitted for further health care was reported in Bijapur. However, here one could note that creation of new districts might be the reason for fewer children patients reported in Bijapur district, for districts of Koppal and Bagalkot were part of Bijapur district earlier. We also collected information on infants and children deaths. It can be observed from Table 9.4 that there were higher number of infants and children death in districts like Bijapur (170), Kolar (175), Belgaum (150), and Raichur (144), in the year 2005–06 (during the period of survey), the number of infant deaths reported in the remaining districts were less than 90 (2004–05). This information was not available in districts like Bagalkot, Davanagere, Dakshin Kannada, Gadag, Haveri, Hassan, Koppal Shimoga and Udupi.

There are three specific reasons as per the hospital authorities, for non-availability of information on infant deaths. They are: (i) taking away dead infants from the hospitals without informing the authorities concerned, (ii) non-maintenance of information on 0–1 year infant deaths, and (iii) normally for delivery women stay only for a few days, i.e., 3 to 4 days in hospitals. After discharge if infant death occurs at home, they do not inform either the hospital authorities or village accountant/anganavadi workers on these deaths.

Table. 9.4 also shows that the number of child deaths were higher in districts of Chitradurga (260) Mangalore (280), Bidar (250), Dakshin Kannada (280), Gulbarga (203), Bagalkot (205) Bijapur (200) and Bellary (210). However, the number of child deaths was comparatively very low in Haveri (40), Belgaum (53), Uttar Kannada and Tumkur (55) Raichur (58). But during the study period it was observed that the districts of Chickmagalur and Shimoga had registered relatively higher number (90) of child deaths (2004–05). In districts of Dharwad, Mandya, Gadag and Kolar this information is not given by the hospital authority.

Children's Health Care Infrastructure: Modern Medical Facilities

In the study we have tried to focus our view on how children's health care is facilitated by the use of modern equipments like ultra-sound, laser, fibre-optic endoscopy and microscope. We have examined the existing facilities like ambulance service, operation theatre, laboratory system, etc. As per the information provided by the hospital authorities, there were no separate emergency services, operation theatre and laboratory system available for children in all the district hospitals in

Table 9.4

Status of In-Patients and Out-Patients in Children's OPD's in District Hospitals of Karnataka

District	Average no. of patients attended*	Average no. of patients admitted*	No. of infant deaths	Total maternal deliveries	No. of children's death
1	2	3	4	5	6
Bagalkot	90–100	5 to 8	NA**	1380	205
Bellary	80–90	4 to 5	86	2950	210
Belgaum	50–60	5 to 7	150	2778	53
Bidar	200–230	8 to 10	86	2675	250
Bijapur	60–80	2 to 4	170	1352	200
Chamarajnagar	70–85	4 to 6	85	2580	120
Chickmagalur	70–80	4 to 5	80	2010	90
Chitradurga	80–90	6 to 7	85	3080	260
Davanagere	100–120	8 to 10	NA	2280	150
Dharwad	60–70	5 to 6	75	2050	nil
Dakshin Kannada	90–100	7 to 8	NA	3210	280
Gadag	60–70	6 to 7	NA	1250	N.A
Gulbarga	85–100	5 to 7	31	2286	203

Cont'd...

Cont'd...

Haveri	30–40	5 to 6	NA	1380	40
Hassan	80–90	4 to 5	NA	2850	186
Kolar	180–200	10 to 12	175		
Koppal	60–80	4 to 5	NA	1475	86
Kodagu	70–80	4 to 6	86	2080	150
Mandya	60–70	5 to 7	346		
Mysore	80–90	6 to8	80	3250	175
Raichur	100–120	8 to 10	144	2300	58
Shimoga	60–70	4 to 6	NA	1850	80
Tumkur	180–200	8–10	51	3050	55
Udupi	80–90	4 to 6	NA	2540	90
Uttar Kannada	50–60	4 to 6	45	1450	55

Source: Field survey during February-March 2006.

Note: Per day ** At the time of delivery, if infant death occurs, the parents take the baby away without taking permission from hospital authority.

Karnataka. These services are common for both adults and children.

In a modern technological society like ours, there is a need to know how modern medical check-up is carried out by using ultra-sound, laser, fibre-optic endoscopy and microscope etc. In this context, an effort has been made to understand whether such infrastructure was provided or not in the respective district hospitals.

It can be observed from Table 9.5 that modern medical check-up by using 'ultra-sound' used for diagnostic purpose was found in all the district hospitals except Bagalkot and Mandya.

Table 9.5 also presents another modern medical facility namely the 'laser' which has got many uses in the medical field such as phototherapy, eye and brain surgery, and other aspects of surgery. As per the information obtained during the time of survey, this medical facility was not provided in majority of the district hospitals like Belgaum, Bidar, Bijapur, Chickmagalur, Chitradurga, Dharwad, Gadag, Gulbarga, Haveri, Kolar, Koppal, Mandya and Raichur. Rest of the district hospitals had this facility and extended health service for children and adults.

The medical equipment called 'fibre-optic endoscopy' is used extensively for both diagnostic and therapeutic purpose. The study found that only 10 districts (Bellary, Chamarajnagar, Davanagere, Dakshin Kannada, Hassan, Kodagu, Mysore, Shimoga and Tumkur) out of 27 had this facility (Table 9.5).

The other medical equipment 'microscope' is an instrument used for producing enlarged images of small objects. It has been provided in almost 50 per cent (12) of the district hospitals. Districts like Chamarajnagar, Chickmagalur, Chitradurga, Dharwad, Gadag, Haveri, Hassan, Koppal, Kodagu, Mandya, Shimoga and Udupi were

Table 9.5

Children Health Care Infrastructure in District Hospitals of Karnataka

District	*Ambulance service*	*Operation theatre*	*Laboratory system*	*X-ray*	*Modern equipments*			
					Ultrasound	*Laser*	*Fibre-optic endoscopy*	*Micro scope*
Bagalkot	Y	Y	Y	Y	N	Y	N	Y
Bellary	Y	Y	Y	Y	Y	Y	Y	Y
Belgaum	Y	Y	Y	Y	Y	N	N	Y
Bidar	Y	Y	Y	Y	Y	N	N	Y
Bijapur	Y	Y	Y	Y	Y	N	N	Y
Chamarajnagar	Y	Y	Y	Y	Y	Y	Y	N
Chickmagalur	Y	Y	Y	Y	Y	Y	N	N
Chitradurga	Y	Y	Y	Y	Y	Y	N	N
Davanagere	Y	Y	Y	Y	Y	Y	Y	Y
Dharwad	Y	Y	Y	Y	Y	Y	N	N
Dakshin Kannada	Y	Y	Y	Y	Y	Y	Y	Y
Gadag	Y	Y	Y	Y	Y	Y	N	N

Cont'd...

Cont'd...

Gulbarga	Y	Y	Y	Y	Y	N	N	Y
Haveri	Y	Y	Y	Y	Y	Y	N	N
Hassn	Y	Y	Y	Y	Y	Y	Y	N
Kolar	N	Y	Y	Y	Y	N	N	Y
Koppal	Y	Y	Y	Y	Y	Y	N	N
Kodagu	Y	Y	Y	Y	Y	Y	Y	N
Mandya	N	N	N	N	N	N	N	N
Mysore	Y	Y	Y	Y	Y	Y	Y	Y
Raichur	Y	Y	Y	Y	Y	N	N	Y
Shimoga	Y	Y	Y	Y	Y	Y	Y	N
Tumkur	Y	Y	Y	Y	Y	N	Y	Y
Udupi	Y	Y	Y	Y	Y	Y	Y	N
Uttar Kannada	Y	Y	Y	Y	Y	Y	Y	Y

Source: Field survey during February-March 2006, Y=Yes and N=No.

not found having this medical facility in their district hospitals during the survey. Further, it has been reported that there were good number of imported medical equipments in the district hospital of Tumkur. However, as operators were not appointed, these medical equipments remained unused.

Children's Health Care Infrastructure Index for Karnataka

To assess public health care infrastructure for children, Children's Health Care Infrastructure Index (CHCII) is prepared by employing a suitable methodology. In Karnataka, health care indicators like children wards, bed strength, number of working doctors, special health care services like neo-natal incentive care (NICU), well-baby clinic and health care facilities provided by modern medical equipments like ultra-sound, microscope etc., in the district hospitals have been considered in developing CHCII for the state of Karnataka by districts.

The scoring orders have been assigned to selected individual factors as shown in Annexure 16. Through the index of the total scoring, the districts have been divided into three groups: (i) districts with relatively good health care infrastructure, (scoring 9 to 12), (ii) districts with relatively moderate scores (5 to 8), and (iii) those with low scores (below 4).

As per the scoring index, the districts of Davanagere, Dakshin Kannada, Mysore, Bellary, Gulbarga, Belgaum, Kolar and Uttar Kannada have relatively good health care infrastructure for children; districts of Bidar, Chitradurga, Dharwad, Hassan, Kodagu, Raichur, Shimoga, Udupi, Chamarajnagar, Chickmagalur, Gadag and Mandya have relatively moderate health care infrastructure, while the newly constituted districts of Bagalkot, Koppal, Haveri and Bijapur have relatively low health care infrastructure for children.

To analyse health care infrastructure, the proportion of child population ranks by districts have been taken into account. The districts have been grouped into High (First order of ranks 1–5), Medium (Second order of ranks 5–10), and Low (Third order of ranks 11–15) based on the ranking obtained. As per the grouping, most of the districts in the northern region (Gulbarga, Koppal, Raichur, Bagalkot, Bidar, Bijapur, Bellary and Belgaum) have high proportion of child population; the districts of Haveri, Gadag, Dharwad, Davanagere, Chitradurga and Kolar have medium proportion of child population, while the remaining districts of Uttar Kannada, Shimoga, Kodagu, Chickmagalur, Mysore, Chamarajnagar, Dakshin Kannada, Hassan, Mandya and Udupi have low proportion of child population.

A detailed analysis of child health care infrastructure has been attempted with a view to linking it up with child health care infrastructure index (Annexure 17) and the proportion of child population (Annexure 18) in Karnataka by districts.

A study on health care infrastructure for children in Karnataka could identify seven different groups of districts based on the indicators of health status as given below:

1. Districts with low health care infrastructure and high proportion of child population (Bagalkot, Bijapur, Haveri and Koppal).
2. Districts with moderate health care infrastructure and high proportion of child population (Bidar and Raichur).
3. Districts with relatively good health care infrastructure and high proportion of child population (Gulbarga, Belgaum and Bellary).
4. Districts with relatively good health care infrastructure and low proportion of child population (Dakshin Kannada, Mysore and Uttar Kannada)

5. Districts with good health care infrastructure with medium proportion of child population (Davanagere and Kolar).
6. Districts with moderate health care infrastructure and medium proportion of child population (Chitradurga, Dharwad and Gadag).
7. The districts with moderate health care infrastructure and low proportion of child population (Hassan, Kodagu, Shimoga, Udupi, Chamarajnagar, Chickmagalur, Mandya and Tumkur).

10

Summary and Conclusions

Karnataka, being one of the progressive states of India, had seen sizeable progress in all spheres of socio-economic development. The early arrival of hydroelectric power generation and industrial growth particularly in southern part had given a head start to economic growth and urban development in the state. After the seventies, growth of tertiary activities not only in the south but even in headquarter towns of taluks and districts have been giving a big push to urban growth with persisting natural hazards in South India, and the impact of globalization and economic liberalization on macro-economic activity in the state have jointly triggered of unhealthy urban growth in the state, particularly in and around big cities like Bangalore, Mysore, Mangalore, Hubli-Dharwad, Belgaum etc.

India has witnessed a major demographic shift in the last quarter of 20th century. The same has been experienced in the state of Karnataka. It is evident that out of 164 taluks there were about 29.26 per cent of taluks which had very high level growth rate of population in the decade 1991–2001. This proportion was 52 per cent in the preceding decade. The industrial district of Shimoga, the coastal districts of Uttar Kannada and Hassan had registered low level growth rate of rural population in the decade 1981–1991. But by the decade

1991–2001 the low level growth rate taluks had concentrated across the state in Karnataka which is evident in the districts of Shimoga, Uttar Kannada, Tumkur, Dharwad, Haveri, Chickmagalur and Mandya. The study finds that there was no significant growth of urban population in Karnataka excepting the taluks in Bangalore, Mysore, Hubli-Dharwad, Belgaum, Shimoga and Mangalore. On the other hand there is a significant growth of rural population in districts of Chickmagalur, Kodagu, Hassan and Shimoga.

All taluks in the northern districts of Raichur, Koppal and Dakshin Kannada, had very high level growth rates in the decade 1981–1991. But by the decade 1991–2001 the concentration of very high (VH) level taluks had witnessed across the districts of Bijapur, Haveri, Raichur, Koppal and Dakshin Kannada. The concentration of very high growth of urban population taluks were higher in the southern region compared to northern region. As is evident by the study, the southern and coastal regions had higher growth of population due to migration and economic expansion. On the other hand northern and central region had higher size population due to higher fertility and low socio-economic development.

About 45.34 per cent of taluks (86) declined to H level from VH level growth rate by the decade 1991–2001, which indicated a marginally slow growth of population in taluks of Karnataka between the decade 1981–1991 and 1991–2001. This constituted a major change in the pattern of population growth in taluks of Karnataka. The number of VH level population growth was high in number in districts like Bijapur, Bagalkot, Bellary, Bidar, Gulbarga, Raichur and Koppal. Between 1981–1991 and 1991–2001 the rural population growth decreased from 15 to 11 per cent. Progress in health and family welfare programmes in the state has influenced to a great extent the increasing trend in medium level and decreasing trend in VH level taluks.

The efforts of the Department of Health and Family Welfare both at the state and central levels have influenced significantly in the reduction of fertility. For instance, the percentage of VH level growth rate taluks in rural population decreased from 46.95 to 18.9. This goes to testifies that some kind of development had indeed taken place in Karnataka. The industrial district of Shimoga, the coastal district of Uttar Kannada and the district of Hassan registered low level growth rate of rural population in the decade 1981–1991. But by the decade 1991–2001, the low level growth rate taluks concentrated across the state in districts like Davanagere, Tumkur, Dharwad, Haveri, Chickmagalur, Mandya including Shimoga, Uttar Kannada and Hassan districts had joined the group of low growth rate taluks.

Except the taluks of Raichur district there was hardly any VH level growth rate of rural population taluks in the decade 1991–2001. Further during 1991–2001, 21 out of 27 districts in Karnataka had shown a declining trend in the number of taluks of high growth rate in rural population. Approximately 66 per cent of the 77 VH taluks in the state declined in their growth rates from VH to H, M or L levels.

The study reveals that modern agriculture was the cause for the higher growth of rural population in taluks like Malur, Chikkaballapur, Athani, Raibagh etc. Similarly, expansion of plantation and estate agriculture in Malnad region in the districts of Shimoga, Kodagu and Hassan resulted in the emergence of VH level taluks in both the decades of 1981–1991 and 1991–2001. Influx of poor and illiterate labour to this region is considerable, and the main reason for this change.

Owing to the industrial development in southern part of the state, the size of urban population is higher in this region as compared to the other regions in the state. Employment opportunities and pull of trade and commerce seem to have influenced to a great extent, rural-urban migration in the districts of Mangalore, Mysore, Belgaum and Dharwad.

In recent times, change in the growth rate of urban population in Karnataka was not significant but, there has been a continuous rise in urban population in some taluks like Bangalore, Mysore, Hubli-Dharwad, Belgaum, Shimoga, and Mangalore due to urbanization. Development of agriculture and irrigation through adoption of modern technology has led to significant growth of rural population in districts like Chickmagalur, Kodagu, Hassan and Shimoga. The share of VH taluks was higher (81%) in southern parts of the state than other regions. Early opening of educational institutions, growth of power and industrial development etc., have largely influenced the higher growth of urban population of southern part in the state.

Northern districts of Raichur, Koppal and Dakshin Kannada had 100 per cent of VH level taluks of the total. But by the decade 1991–2001, concentration of VH level taluks had moved across districts of Chitradurga, Bijapur, Haveri, Bidar, Raichur, Koppal and Dakshin Kannada districts. This is mainly due to developmental initiatives taken on the one hand, and migration of rural population to urban areas on the other. Twenty-seven out of 99 taluks had shown decline in their growth rate from VH to H level by the decade 1991–2001. Due to growing urbanization in the state about 20 new taluks moved to VH level growth rate from medium and low levels, which points to significant growth of urban population. Thus, by the year 2002, there were a large numbers of taluks in VH level in the growth rate of urban population as compared to rural population.

Development of irrigation in Hosanagar and Sorab taluks in Shimoga district, opening of Hemavathi canal irrigation in Turuvekere taluk of Tumkur district and expansion of plantation agriculture in Hassan district, have influenced to some extent, the demotion of some taluks from VH to H and low level in the growth rate of urban population.

This does not include the displacement of population from rural areas or even urban areas to big cities in the state.

In Karnataka, the districts of Bidar, Bellary, Bijapur, Gulbarga, and Raichur were identified as high-fertility districts. But, across these districts, there were disparities in regard to growth pattern across taluks in a district as also across taluks in different districts. However taluks like Basavakalyana, Bidar and Homnabad in Bidar district, Bellary, Hospet, Kudligi, Sandur, Siruguppa and H.B. Hally in Bellary district, Bijapur and Basavana Bagevadi in Bijapur district, Afzalpur, Chicholli, Chitapur, Gulbarga, Jevargi, Shahapur, Shorapur, Yadgir and Sedam, in Gulbarga district, Devadurga, Lingasugur, Manvi, Raichur, Sindanur and Gangavathi, in Raichur district all have recorded sizeable growth of population during the decade under review.

Hence, there is a need to give special attention to these taluks for combating population growth. What is needed is to formulate policies and plans for socio-economic development, particularly of weaker sections (minorities). In fact, weaker sections are migrating to bigger urban areas across state in search of livelihood. Sustainable agricultural practices, water harvesting, compulsory people participation in literacy etc., are some of the areas of development which can be initiated in these taluks as remedial measures.

The overall growth of female child population in Karnataka was absolutely negative in the decade 1991–2001. And further there was a significant decline in the growth of female child population in the district of Bijapur, Dharwad and Chitradurga. In this circumstance one can predict that if the current rate of decline in female child population continues in these districts there will be a severe shortage of girls of marriageable age in future. Hence, there is a need to correct the gender imbalance through appropriate steps.

The study found that one or the other problems have been drawn attention in the district hospitals. Sixteen out of 53 sanctioned posts of pediatrics were vacant in district hospitals of Karnataka. There is also need to provide modern medical equipment to the hospitals to diagnose the heath problems. To streamline these problems the department of health and family welfare must address the issues through auditing.

Districts in the southern region have low proportion of child population, while the opposite is the case in the districts in the northern region. Proportion of female child population in total population in Karnataka was higher than that of male child population in 1981, which declined by the year 2001. In the decade 1981–1991, overall growth rate of child population in Karnataka was 8.5 per cent; the rate of growth was negative in the decade 1991–2001. There has been a drastic change in the growth rate of child population in Karnataka by districts in two decades under review. Economically backward districts of Gulbarga and Raichur have registered very high growth rate of child population even in the decade 1991–2001.

Most of the districts in southern region have registered negative rate of growth in child population in the decade 1991–2001, and excepting, Belgaum, Gulbarga and Bangalore Urban no other district witnessed any significant growth in child population in the state. The growth of male child population in Karnataka increased from 20.4 per cent in the decade 1981–1991 to 44.4 per cent in the decade 1991–2001. The growth of male child population was much higher than the growth of female child population during the decade between 1981–1991 and 1991–2001. In the decade 1991–2001, all districts in Karnataka excepting Chitradurga and Dharwad, reported a positive growth in male child population; Bangalore Urban district recorded the highest growth.

The percentage change in male child population between two decades was highest in Bangalore Urban. A drastic decline was seen in the growth of female child population in the decade 1991–2001. Between the two decades (1981–1991 and 1991–2001) the rate of negative growth of female child population in Karnataka was highest in the district of Dharwad, Bijapur, Raichur and Chitradurga. The growth rate of female child population was absolutely negative in most of the districts of southern region in the decade 1991–2001. Except Bangalore Urban and Gulbarga, no districts reported a positive growth in female child population in the decade 1991–2001.

As per 2001 census, ST population constitutes about 8.8 per cent of the total population of India. The growth rate variation between two decades of ST population was minus 6 per cent. The proportion of ST rural population has declined to 84.23 per cent in 2001 from 92.6 per cent in 1991. On the other hand urban population increased from 7.4 per cent in 1991 to 15.77 per cent in 2001. Three-fourth's of ST population has been residing in the north and north-eastern region in the country. A remarkable change in the growth of ST population across states was noticed in the decade 1991–2001. The overall growth of ST total population has come down from 24.85 per cent in the decade 1981–1991 to 18.58 per cent in the decade 1991–2001.

The progressive state of Karnataka has ranked first (44.70%) in terms of ST population growth in India, in the decade the highest rate of ST total population growth registered in Karnataka. The states like Nagaland, Manipur, Meghalaya, Mizoram, Uttar Pradesh and union territory of Dadra Nagar Haveli had higher rate of growth with above the national average of 18.58 per cent in the decade 1991–2001. The growth rate of STs between the decades was absolutely negative at national level. Excepting the states of Karnataka, Daman & Diu, Bihar, Tamil Nadu, Himachal Pradesh,

Nagaland, and Arunachal Pradesh no other state showed a positive growth rate of their absolute population.

There was a considerable reduction (13%) of rural population growth between the decades under consideration. In the respect of rural population growth of Scheduled Tribes in India, the rate of growth was completely positive with higher rates of 41.06 per cent in the decade 1991–2001 and again its ranked first in the country. There has been significant growth of ST rural population in Lakshdweep, Mizoram, Dadra & Nagar Haveli, Bihar, Himachal Pradesh and Tamil Nadu in the decade 1991–2001 as compared to the previous decade. The overall growth rate of rural ST declined from 23.80 per cent in the decade 1991–2001 to 10.49 per cent in the decade 1981–1991.

The decadal growth of urban population of STs in India was reduced from 37.87 per cent in the decade 1981–1991 to 27.81 per cent in the decade 1991–2001. The states of Karnataka, Uttar Pradesh, and Tamil Nadu had registered the growth rate above the national average of 27.81 per cent. Further, the growth of ST urban population was highest in Daman & Diu, Uttar Pradesh, and Karnataka and their rate of growth was 64.18 per cent, 39.85, and 45.95 per cent respectively. On the other hand southern state of Kerala, West Bengal, Mizoram and Maharashtra have paid greater attention with declined growth of urban population in the decade 1991–2001 as compared to previous decade.

During the study period, there were no permanent doctors at COPDs in district hospitals of Bagalkot, Haveri, Koppal and Bijapur. These districts have medical colleges and derived benefits from the health care provided by house surgeons (trainee doctors). The study found that the temporary doctors on contract basis working in the hospitals of Belgaum, Davanagere, Dakshin Kannada, Gulbarga and Mysore. Sixteen out of 53 posts of pediatrics were vacant in children's hospitals in the district hospitals in Karnataka. Most of which comes in the northern region. Higher number of beds was found in children's wards in district hospitals of Gulbarga, Davanagere, Mysore and Dakshin Kannada. The special ward called NICU was not in existence in hospitals of Bidar, Bijapur, Chamarajnagar, Gadag, Haveri, Kolar, Koppal and Udupi.

On an average, 200–300 patients were found coming for health check-up in a day at the COPD in the district hospital of Bidar. This number is found to be the highest in the state. A higher number of in-patients per day were found seeking admission for health care in the hospitals of Kolar, Bidar, Davanagere and Raichur. As per the information collected by the study, a higher number of infant and children deaths were reported in the hospitals of Chitradurga, Mangalore, Bidar, Dakshin Kannada, Gulbarga, Bagalkot, Bijapur and Bellary. The modern medical equipments like ultrasound were found in all the hospitals, excepting Bagalkot and Mandya. A majority of district hospitals did not have laser equipment.

Out of 25 districts in Karnataka, only ten district hospitals were found having fibre-optic endoscope for use in both diagnostic and therapeutic procedures. Thirteen out of 27 district hospitals in Karnataka had been provided with microscope for use in laboratories. Out of 25 districts in Karnataka only 10 district hospitals had fiber-optic endoscope used extensively for both diagnostic and therapeutic purpose. Around 13 out of 27 hospitals had modern medical service of microscope.

Although, the districts like Bagalkot, Haveri, Koppal and Bijapur were newly constituted districts, yet, with characteristic constraints for the smooth functioning of the COPD, there is a need to fill-up the vacant posts of children's doctors immediately. Sixteen out of 53 sanctioned posts of pediatrics were vacant in district hospitals in Karnataka, though most of the weaker sections and also general people depend on health services by these district hospitals. In this context this matter should draw government's attention speedily, and the government should take immediate remedial steps in the matter. Upgrading services like increasing children's ward and also bed strength etc., need to be done by the public health care department of the government. At present, proportion of child population varies across districts in Karnataka. In this context, the study finds that there is a need to increase bed strength in children's wards according to the proportion of child population in the state. Also, there is a need to build neo-natal incentive care units in the hospitals of Bidar, Bijapur, Chamarajangar, Haveri, Kolar, Koppal and Udupi.

The higher number of child patients coming for health check-up per day in hospitals of Kolar, Bidar, Davanagere and Raichur, necessitates commensurate increase in health care facilities there. There is also a need to provide modern medical equipment, i.e., ultrasound for the hospitals of Bagalkot and Mandya. The majority of the hospitals in districts need to have laser machine for health check-up. Out of 25 districts in Karnataka, only 10 district hospitals have fibre-optic endoscope. It is, therefore, necessary to provide this equipment to the district hospitals. These are the suggestions for further streamlining of children out-patient departments (COPD) and to improve health care infrastructure in the district hospitals of Karnataka. The findings of the study can be taken note of and implemented by the Department of Health and Family Welfare, Government of Karnataka.

Last but not the least, the government's efforts in controlling population growth in Karnataka during the last two decades have indeed brought about a decline in the rate of child population growth. Further, it also registered a negative rate of growth. From this we can infer that this was due to the progressive steps adopted by the state of Karnataka. The overall growth of female child population in

Karnataka was absolutely negative in the decade 1991–2001, and there was a significant decline in the growth rate of female child population in districts of Bijapur, Dharwad and Chitradurga. If current rate of decline in female child population continues in these districts, there will be a disturbing imbalance in sex-ratios, and in future, there might be severe shortage of girls of marriageable age. Hence, there is a need to correct the gender imbalance through appropriate steps.

Overall, during the past 20 years there has been a continuous fertility decline in India. The same trend is evident in Karnataka also. Disparity in socio-economic development indicators has been growing between northern and southern region of Karnataka. The districts in southern region have been more successful in controlling population growth, with the result; most of the districts in northern region have a higher rate of growth in their child population as compared to that of southern region. The districts of Gulbarga and Raichur have recorded high rate of growth in child population, and it was much higher than the other districts in the state. To control the situation, the governments must take this issue from a demographic point of view through programmes and policy measures. Special care has to be taken by providing public health care and urban amenities to rural population in these districts through hobly or grama panchayathi level institutions. Otherwise this will retard the further growth and development of the region. It is necessary to create awareness and ensure participation of masses to bring about population reduction.

Annexures

Annexure 1

Decadal Population Growth by Taluks in Karnataka 1981–1991 and 1991–2001

District	S. No.	Taluk	Total 1981–91	Total 1991–2001	Increase(+) Decrease(–)	Rank in 1981–91	Rank in 1991–2001
1	2	3	4	5	6	7	8
		I. Bangalore division					
1. Chitradurga	1	Challakere(1)	21.61	16.03	–5.58	17	37
	2	Chitradurga(1)	18.98	14.47	–4.51	39	49
	3	Hiriyur(1)	14.21	13.61	–0.61	91	59
	4	Holalakere(1)	11.94	9.38	–2.55	121	120
	5	Hosadurga(1)	13.42	8.93	–4.49	102	125
	6	Molakalmur(1)	20.51	18.31	–2.20	27	16
2. Davanagere	1	Davanagere(2)	21.50	14.66	–6.84	19	47
	2	Harihara(2)	20.05	11.75	–8.30	31	86
	3	Channagiri(2)	13.42	12.01	–1.41	102	82
	4	Honnalli(2)	13.86	10.14	–3.72	94	108
	5	Harapanahally(2)	21.57	12.91	–8.66	18	66
	6	Jagalur(2)	18.65	13.92	–4.72	43	58
3. Kolar	1	Bagepally(3)	12.75	14.02	1.27	109	56
	2	Bangarpet(3)	12.06	7.97	–4.08	120	136
	3	Chikkaballpur(3)	17.04	11.45	–5.59	60	93
	4	Chintamani(3)	15.73	13.11	–2.62	73	65
	5	Gauribidanoor(3)	10.85	11.44	0.59	130	94
	6	Gudibanda(3)	14.22	11.59	–2.63	90	90
	7	Kolar(3)	13.78	17.08	3.30	95	28
	8	Malur(3)	16.87	16.01	–0.85	64	38
	9	Mulbagil(3)	15.88	12.28	–3.59	72	77
	10	Sidlagatta(3)	14.18	13.26	–0.92	92	64
	11	Srinivaspur(3)	12.27	11.65	–0.62	115	88
4. Shimoga	1	Badravathi(4)	11.23	4.22	–7.01	128	153
	2	Hosanagar(4)	1.37	10.68	9.31	150	103

Cont'd...

Cont'd...

	3	Sagar(4)	9.53	11.86	2.33	138	85
	4	Shikaripur(4)	18.63	11.63	–7.00	44	89
	5	Shimoga(4)	19.85	17.90	–1.95	34	20
	6	Sorab(4)	13.59	12.50	–1.08	99	74
	7	Tirthahally(4)	4.68	8.47	3.79	149	130
5. Tumkur	1	C.N.Hally(5)	11.19	7.73	–3.46	129	138
	2	Gubbi(5)	13.68	9.67	–4.01	98	116
	3	Koratagere(5)	12.10	9.56	–2.54	119	118
	4	Kunigal(5)	11.24	0.42	–10.83	127	155
	5	Madhugiri(5)	12.76	7.63	–5.13	108	139
	6	Pavagada(5)	13.72	13.60	–0.12	96	60
	7	Sira(5)	16.05	15.34	–0.71	71	45
	8	Tiptur(5)	10.57	9.81	–0.76	132	115
	9	Tumkur(5)	21.57	17.52	–4.05	18	24
	10	Turuvekere(5)	10.03	5.56	–4.47	137	150
		II Belgaum division					
6. Belgaum	1	Athani(6)	86.24	17.24	–68.99	1	26
	2	Belgaum(6)	18.33	17.15	–1.18	47	27
	3	Chhikkodi(6)	13.41	14.09	0.68	103	54
	4	Gokak(6)	18.53	16.11	–2.42	46	36
	5	Hukkeri(6)	11.84	13.59	1.75	123	61
	6	Khanapur(6)	14.43	10.88	–3.55	88	99
	7	Parasgad(6)	18.74	12.04	–6.70	41	81
	8	Raibagh(6)	24.73	18.60	–6.13	7	13
	9	Ramadurga(6)	17.46	10.63	–6.83	52	105
	10	Sampagon(6)	17.00	12.71	–4.30	62	69
7. Bijapur	1	Basavana b.wadi(7)	14.43	15.22	0.80	88	46
	2	Bijapur(7)	19.90	16.91	–2.99	33	30
	3	Indi(7)	19.42	14.37	–5.05	36	50
	4	Muddebihal (7)	15.68	13.56	–2.12	74	62
	5	Sindgi(7)	20.72	14.00	–6.72	23	57

Cont'd...

Cont'd...

8. Bagalkote	1	Badami(8)	16.32	12.09	-4.22	72	80
	2	Bagalkot(8)	12.72	15.46	2.75	110	43
	3	Bilgi(8)	17.43	16.20	-1.24	53	35
	4	Hungund(8)	10.24	14.55	4.31	135	48
	5	Jamkhandi(8)	20.16	16.91	-3.24	30	30
	6	Mudhol(8)	15.50	20.37	4.86	80	8
9. Dharwad	1	Dharwad(9)	16.93	11.93	-5.01	63	83
	2	Kalgatgi(9)	17.93	11.51	-6.42	49	92
	3	Kundgol(9)	7.57	12.16	4.60	145	79
	4	Hubli(9)	14.44	11.91	-2.53	87	84
	5	Navalgund(9)	14.48	8.59	-5.89	86	127
10. Gadag	1	Mundargi(10)	14.02	12.48	-1.54	93	75
	2	Naragund(10)	21.00	6.46	-14.54	22	144
	3	Ron(10)	12.30	10.77	-1.53	113	102
	4	Shirhatti(10)	12.80	12.83	0.04	107	68
	5	Gadag(10)	12.28	12.68	0.40	114	70
11. Haveri	1	Hangal(11)	16.60	11.42	-5.18	66	95
	2	Haveri(11)	17.59	12.63	-4.96	51	71
	3	Hirekerur(11)	15.48	9.65	-5.83	81	117
	4	Byadgi(11)	16.55	12.51	-4.04	67	73
	5	Ranibennur(11)	18.73	11.71	-7.01	42	87
	6	Savanur(11)	15.52	14.05	-1.48	79	55
	7	Shiggon(11)	17.39	11.54	-5.85	54	91
12. Uttar Kannada	1	Ankola(12)	11.23	10.08	-1.15	128	109
	2	Bhatkal(12)	24.90	13.61	-11.29	6	59
	3	Haliyal(12)	-40.47	10.85	-29.62	153	100
	4	Honnavar(12)	12.24	9.04	-3.21	116	124
	5	Karwar(12)	10.44	5.14	-5.30	133	151
	6	Kumta(12)	12.54	8.01	-4.53	112	135
	7	Mundgol(12)	21.72	17.29	-4.43	15	25
	8	Siddapur(12)	7.77	9.14	1.37	143	122
	9	Sirsi(12)	11.66	12.88	1.23	124	67

Cont'd...

Cont'd...

		III Gulbarga division					
13. Bellary	1	Bellary(13)	22.09	20.79	−1.29	13	5
	2	Hadagali(13)	21.62	12.38	−9.24	16	76
	3	H.B. Hally(13)	26.82	15.55	−11.27	3	42
	4	Hospet(13)	15.60	16.55	0.94	76	32
	5	Kudaligi(13)	24.51	19.36	−5.15	8	12
	6	Sandur(13)	19.02	18.18	−0.84	38	18
	7	Siruguppa(13)	21.39	19.50	−1.88	20	11
14. Bidar	1	Aurad(14)	17.26	14.37	−2.89	56	50
	2	Basavakalyna(14)	18.74	17.86	−0.88	41	21
	3	Bhalki(14)	18.24	13.28	−4.97	48	63
	4	Bidar(14)	25.21	18.27	−6.94	5	17
	5	Homnabad(14)	21.83	16.82	−5.01	14	32
15. Gulbarga	1	Afzalpur(15)	17.09	16.22	−0.86	59	34
	2	Aland(15)	17.15	12.22	−4.93	58	78
	3	Chincholli(15)	16.37	15.42	−0.95	69	44
	4	Chitapur(15)	16.67	15.63	−1.05	65	41
	5	Gulbarga(15)	23.18	22.46	−0.72	11	2
	6	Jevargi(15)	18.90	19.79	0.89	40	10
	7	Sedam(15)	20.67	16.82	−3.85	24	31
	8	Shahapur(15)	20.21	18.16	−2.05	28	19
	9	Shorapur(15)	20.66	16.34	−4.33	25	33
	10	Yadgir(15)	18.56	15.90	−2.66	45	39
16. Raichur	1	Devadurga(16)	20.17	20.48	0.32	29	7
	2	Lingasugur(16)	23.63	18.38	−5.25	10	15
	3	Manvi(16)	25.24	18.58	−6.66	4	14
	4	Raichur(16)	23.65	17.58	−6.07	9	23
	5	Sindanoor(16)	23.11	20.94	−2.17	12	4
	6	Gangavathi(16)	19.73	21.15	1.42	35	3
17. Koppal	1	Koppal(17)	20.62	19.85	−0.77	26	9
	2	Kustagi(17)	27.92	20.66	−7.27	2	6
	3	Yelbarga(17)	21.29	17.05	−4.24	21	29

Cont'd...

Cont'd...

		IV Mysore division					
18. Chickma-galur	1	Chickmagalur(18)	10.16	14.16	4.00	136	53
	2	Kadur(18)	10.82	10.19	–0.62	131	107
	3	Koppa(18)	6.10	8.18	2.08	147	131
	4	Mudigere(18)	11.64	9.18	–2.47	125	121
	5	N.R.Pura(18)	8.71	14.19	5.48	140	52
	6	Sringeri(18)	4.95	9.91	4.96	148	114
	7	Tarikere(18)	12.30	8.54	–3.75	113	128
19. Dakshin Kannada	1	Bantval(19)	11.92	10.66	–1.26	122	104
	2	Belthangadi(19)	17.01	14.24	–2.77	61	51
	3	Mangalore(19)	12.59	23.96	11.37	111	1
	4	Puttur(19)	17.30	10.84	–6.46	55	101
	5	Sulya(19)	15.57	11.32	–4.26	78	97
20. Udupi	1	Karkal(20)	8.33	35.70	–44.03	142	156
	2	Kundapur(20)	11.23	6.82	–4.41	128	143
	3	Udupi(20)	7.13	6.32	–0.81	146	146
21. Hassan	1	Alur(21)	12.17	8.12	–4.05	118	133
	2	Arkalgud(21)	15.22	8.66	–6.57	83	126
	3	Arasikere(21)	10.25	6.16	–4.09	134	148
	4	Belur(21)	13.15	7.31	–5.84	104	141
	5	Channaraya(21)	14.21	8.59	–5.62	91	127
	6	Hassan(21)	15.67	12.59	–3.08	75	72
	7	Holenarsipur(21)	17.24	9.49	–7.75	57	119
	8	Sakaleshpur(21)	8.61	7.14	–1.47	141	142
22. Kodagu	1	Madikeri(22)	7.61	10.28	2.67	144	106
	2	Somavarpet(22)	10.24	11.36	1.12	135	96
	3	Virajpet(22)	–1.02	10.00	8.98	151	110
23. Mandaya	1	Krishnarajpet(23)	15.58	10.93	–4.65	77	98
	2	Maddur(23)	13.53	2.77	–10.76	100	154
	3	Malavalli(23)	13.12	6.29	–6.83	106	147
	4	Mandya(23)	13.51	5.57	–7.94	101	149

Cont'd...

Cont'd...

	5	Nagamangala(23)	11.56	6.35	–5.21	126	145
	6	Pandavapura(23)	14.93	8.49	–6.44	84	129
	7	Srirangapatna(23)	10.03	9.97	–0.07	137	113
24. Mysore	1	H.D.Kote(24)	20.02	12.01	–8.01	32	82
	2	Hunsur(24)	19.27	12.50	–6.77	37	74
	3	Krishnarajnag(24)	15.44	9.13	–6.31	82	123
	4	Mysore(24)	24.51	17.72	–6.79	8	22
	5	Nanjangud(24)	16.43	10.00	–6.43	68	110
	6	Piriyapatna(24)	17.90	15.76	–2.13	50	40
	7	T.narasipur(24)	14.64	7.49	–7.15	85	140
25. Chamarajnagar	1	Chamarajnagar(25)	11.56	6.35	–5.21	126	145
	2	Gundlupet(25)	13.71	8.15	–5.55	97	132
	3	Kollegal(25)	13.13	9.56	–3.56	105	118
	4	Yelndur(25)	14.42	8.02	–6.39	89	134
Karnataka			21.12	17.25	–3.87	—	—

Annexure 2

Decadal Rural Population Growth in Karnataka by Taluks for the Decade 1981–1991 and 1991–2001

District	S. No.	Taluk	Decade 1981–1991	Decade 1991–2001	Rank in 1981–1991	Rank in 1991–2001	Increase(+) or Decrease(–)
1	2	3	4	5	6	7	8
		I. Bangalore division					
1. Chitradurga	1	Challakere(1)	19.50	15.03	34	31	–4.47
	2	Chitradurga(1)	14.76	13.03	74	50	–1.74
	3	Hiriyur(1)	10.53	11.45	126	71	0.91
	4	Holalakere(1)	11.37	8.84	116	112	–2.52
	5	Hosadurga(1)	12.02	7.29	112	122	–4.73
	6	Molakalmur(1)	21.08	15.76	24	24	–5.32
2. Davanagere	1	Davanagere(2)	8.73	6.85	136	126	–1.89
	2	Harihara(2)	19.42	4.92	36	137	–14.50
	3	Channagiri(2)	13.27	11.22	95	77	–2.04
	4	Honnalli(2)	14.14	13.53	80	40	–0.61
	5	Harapanahally(2)	21.83	11.87	21	64	–9.96
	6	Jagalur(2)	18.56	13.51	43	42	–5.05
3. Kolar	1	Bagepally(3)	10.62	10.70	124	87	0.08
	2	Bangarpet(3)	13.79	10.50	86	91	–3.29
	3	Chikkaballpur(3)	17.80	10.39	49	92	–7.41
	4	Chintamani(3)	13.97	9.95	84	97	–4.02
	5	Gauribidanoor(3)	8.96	13.51	135	43	4.55
	6	Gudibanda(3)	14.04	11.07	82	81	–2.97
	7	Kolar(3)	10.80	12.20	122	58	1.40
	8	Malur(3)	15.30	14.72	69	34	–0.58
	9	Mulbagil(3)	14.01	10.62	83	89	–3.39
	10	Sidlagatta(3)	16.89	6.41	58	128	–10.48
	11	Srinivaspur(3)	10.85	9.34	121	104	–1.51
4. Shimoga	1	Badravathi(4)	10.15	1.63	129	143	–8.52
	2	Hosanagar(4)	–1.82	13.59	151	39	15.42
	3	Sagar(4)	10.95	12.02	120	58	1.07
	4	Shikaripur(4)	19.49	10.62	35	87	–8.87
	5	Shimoga(4)	18.55	2.10	44	142	–16.45

Cont'd...

Cont'd...

	6	Sorab(4)	13.28	13.51	94	42	0.23
	7	Tirthahally(4)	4.42	8.12	148	113	3.69
5. Tumkur	1	C.N.Hally(5)	11.14	6.13	118	129	–5.01
	2	Gubbi(5)	13.56	9.10	89	104	–4.46
	3	Koratagere(5)	10.57	9.01	125	106	–1.56
	4	Kunigal(5)	10.04	–2.98	130	149	–13.02
	5	Madhugiri(5)	12.33	6.60	108	124	–5.73
	6	Pavagada(5)	12.14	15.68	110	25	3.54
	7	Sira(5)	15.88	11.75	67	64	–4.13
	8	Tiptur(5)	9.46	2.59	131	140	–6.87
	9	Tumkur(5)	8.41	8.02	138	114	–0.39
	10	Turuvekere(5)	8.45	5.20	137	133	–3.25
		II Belgaum division					
6. Belgaum	1	Athani(6)	86.27	16.80	1	17	–69.47
	2	Belgaum(6)	10.29	11.59	128	67	1.30
	3	Chhikkodi(6)	12.55	13.88	104	36	1.33
	4	Gokak(6)	18.76	17.92	42	12	–0.84
	5	Hukkeri(6)	10.44	14.80	127	32	4.36
	6	Khanapur(6)	14.54	11.32	76	72	–3.22
	7	Parasgad(6)	18.52	11.89	45	61	–6.63
	8	Raibagh(6)	25.86	20.03	11	3	–5.83
	9	Ramadurga(6)	19.23	9.00	38	107	–10.23
	10	Sampagon(6)	16.40	11.49	63	68	–4.91
7. Bijapur	1	Basavana b.wadi(7)	14.07	14.79	81	33	0.72
	2	Bijapur(7)	17.26	11.27	54	74	–6.00
	3	Indi(7)	18.52	13.80	45	38	–4.73
	4	Muddebihal (7)	14.50	11.02	77	80	–3.48
	5	Sindgi(7)	21.85	11.44	20	70	–10.41
8. Bagalkote	1	Badami(8)	16.15	12.72	66	50	–3.43
	2	Bagalkot(8)	13.27	15.45	95	29	2.18
	3	Bilgi(8)	25.88	5.96	10	131	–19.92
	4	Hungund(8)	16.50	12.57	61	53	–3.92
	5	Jamkhandi(8)	24.21	16.92	14	16	–7.29
	6	Mudhol(8)	23.39	19.02	18	7	–4.37
9. Dharwad	1	Dharwad(9)	17.49	12.00	51	59	–5.50
	2	Kalgatgi(9)	27.03	0.89	6	145	–26.14

Cont'd...

Cont'd...

	3	Kundgol(9)	8.16	12.10	139	57	3.95
	4	Hubli(9)	14.44	11.91	78	60	–2.53
	5	Navalgund(9)	11.20	9.28	117	102	–1.93
10. Gadag	1	Mundargi(10)	13.31	11.15	91	77	–2.16
	2	Naragund(10)	20.78	5.61	27	132	–15.17
	3	Ron(10)	12.30	9.95	109	95	–2.36
	4	Shirhatti(10)	13.30	13.22	92	46	–0.08
	5	Gadag(10)	12.63	11.85	103	63	–0.78
11. Haveri	1	Hangal(11)	16.41	10.81	62	83	–5.60
	2	Haveri(11)	17.04	10.82	57	82	–6.22
	3	Hirekerur(11)	20.83	2.36	26	141	–18.48
	4	Byadgi(11)	17.39	10.68	53	86	–6.71
	5	Ranibennur(11)	20.36	3.27	29	138	–17.09
	6	Savanur(11)	15.45	13.28	68	44	–2.17
	7	Shiggon(11)	16.31	–4.59	64	151	–20.90
12.Uttar Kannada	1	Ankola(12)	11.44	–3.17	115	150	–14.60
	2	Bhatkal(12)	26.97	9.01	7	106	–17.96
	3	Haliyal(12)	12.46	12.52	107	54	0.06
	4	Honnavar(12)	12.95	9.02	98	105	–3.93
	5	Karwar(12)	1.25	–9.01	150	153	–10.26
	6	Kumta(12)	12.99	3.02	97	139	–9.97
	7	Mundgol(12)	35.49	–0.65	2	147	–36.13
	8	Siddapur(12)	20.09	–5.56	31	152	–25.65
	9	Sirsi(12)	5.72	7.42	146	118	1.69
	10	Supa(12)	–8.85	11.18	155	76	20.03
	11	Yellapur(12)	5.31	8.41	147	111	3.09
		III Gulbarga division					
13.Bellary	1	Bellary(13)	26.24	19.01	9	8	–7.23
	2	Hadagali(13)	20.89	11.13	25	78	–9.76
	3	H.B. Hally(13)	26.82	15.55	8	27	–11.27
	4	Hospet(13)	17.26	18.01	54	11	0.75
	5	Kudaligi(13)	31.98	12.00	3	59	–19.97
	6	Sandur(13)	28.68	–83.43	4	155	–54.75
	7	Siruguppa(13)	20.43	17.51	28	14	–2.93
14.Bidar	1	Aurad(14)	18.55	11.29	44	73	–7.27
	2	Basavakalyna(14)	18.03	15.57	47	26	–2.46

Cont'd...

Cont'd...

	3	Bhalki(14)	16.64	11.67	60	65	–4.96
	4	Bidar(14)	15.07	13.27	71	45	–1.80
	5	Homnabad(14)	23.98	13.81	16	37	–10.16
15.Gulbarga	1	Afzalpur(15)	24.11	6.15	15	127	–17.96
	2	Aland(15)	19.03	10.55	40	88	–8.49
	3	Chincholli(15)	17.25	13.52	55	41	–3.73
	4	Chitapur(15)	18.26	12.40	46	55	–5.86
	5	Gulbarga(15)	14.95	13.20	72	47	–1.75
	6	Jevargi(15)	23.29	12.67	19	51	–10.63
	7	Sedam(15)	12.53	16.75	105	18	4.22
	8	Shahapur(15)	16.67	16.57	59	19	–0.10
	9	Shorapur(15)	18.52	17.13	45	15	–1.39
	10	Yadgir(15)	21.09	13.36	23	43	–7.73
16.Raichur	1	Devadurga(16)	20.16	19.22	30	6	–0.94
	2	Lingasugur(16)	19.30	18.96	37	9	–0.34
	3	Manvi(16)	25.39	17.71	12	13	–7.67
	4	Raichur(16)	15.07	15.92	71	23	0.85
	5	Sindanoor(16)	19.68	19.58	33	5	–0.10
	6	Gangavathi(16)	17.05	21.55	56	1	4.50
17.Koppal	1	Koppal(17)	21.60	20.15	22	2	–1.45
	2	Kustagi(17)	28.62	19.67	5	4	–8.95
	3	Yelbarga(17)	25.14	12.83	13	49	–12.31
		IV Mysore division					
18.Chickma-galur	1	Chickmagalur(18)	13.24	0.72	96	146	–12.51
	2	Kadur(18)	9.38	9.10	132	104	–0.28
	3	Koppa(18)	6.16	8.58	143	110	2.42
	4	Mudigere(18)	12.66	9.38	102	99	–3.28
	5	N.R.Pura(18)	9.01	14.40	134	35	5.39
	6	Sringeri(18)	6.08	10.88	144	81	4.79
	7	Tarikere(18)	13.29	10.10	93	92	–3.18
19. Dakshin Kannada	1	Bantval(19)	9.10	9.22	133	103	0.12
	2	Belthangadi(19)	19.69	11.62	32	66	–8.07
	3	Mangalore(19)	–5.09	18.05	153	10	12.96
	4	Puttur(19)	13.95	6.12	85	130	–7.83
	5	Sulya(19)	23.90	–1.71	17	148	22.19

Cont'd...

Cont'd...

20. Udupi	1	Karkal(20)	7.34	32.44	140	154	–25.10
	2	Kundapur(20)	11.78	16.22	114	20	4.44
	3	Udupi(20)	–8.28	7.02	154	121	–1.26
21. Hassan	1	Alur(21)	11.93	7.28	113	120	–4.65
	2	Arkalgud(21)	15.23	12.64	70	52	–2.60
	3	Arasikere(21)	6.34	7.56	141	117	1.22
	4	Belur(21)	12.48	6.14	106	128	–6.35
	5	Channaraya(21)	13.37	6.95	90	122	–6.42
	6	Hassan(21)	6.20	11.38	142	71	5.19
	7	Holenarsipur(21)	17.77	8.89	50	108	–8.89
	8	Sakaleshpur(21)	3.68	4.76	149	135	1.08
22.Kodagu	1	Madikeri(22)	5.74	9.91	145	96	4.16
	2	Somavarpet(22)	12.09	15.18	111	30	3.10
	3	Virajpet(22)	–2.84	13.27	152	45	10.43
23. Mandaya	1	Krishnarajpet(23)	14.40	10.00	79	94	–4.40
	2	Maddur(23)	12.87	1.38	99	144	–11.49
	3	Malavalli(23)	12.80	7.72	100	115	–5.08
	4	Mandya(23)	12.09	4.25	111	136	–7.84
	5	Nagamangala(23)	10.67	9.35	123	100	–1.31
	6	Pandavapura(23)	15.45	10.08	68	93	–5.37
	7	Srirangapatna(23)	13.78	10.35	87	91	–3.43
24.Mysore	1	H.D.Kote(24)	18.81	16.07	41	21	–2.73
	2	Hunsur(24)	19.10	10.76	39	88	–8.33
	3	Krishnarajnag(24)	13.76	8.29	88	120	–5.48
	4	Mysore(24)	17.46	15.93	52	22	–1.54
	5	Nanjangud(24)	16.20	9.74	65	97	–6.46
	6	Piriyapatna(24)	18.00	15.50	48	28	–2.50
	7	Tirumakudalu Navasipura(24)	14.79	6.28	73	126	–8.51
25.Chamaraj-nagar	1	Chamarajnagar(25)	12.72	3.67	101	137	–9.05
	2	Gundlupet(25)	13.31	8.02	91	114	–5.29
	3	Kollegal(25)	11.09	9.57	119	98	–1.53
	4	Yelndur(25)	14.64	7.71	75	116	0.00
Karnataka			**15.00**	**10.75**	**—**	**—**	**–4.05**

Annexure 3

Decadal Urban Population Growth in Karnataka by Taluks

District	S. No.	Taluk	Decade 1981–91	Decade 1991–2001	Rank in 1981–1991	Rank in 1991–2001	Increase(+) Decrease(–)
1	*2*	*3*	*4*	*5*	*6*	*7*	*8*
		I. Bangalore division					
1.Chitradurga	1	Challakere(1)	34.73	21.80	13	46	–12.93
	2	Chitradurga(1)	27.90	17.36	29	76	–10.53
	3	Hiriyur(1)	32.95	23.15	15	41	–9.80
	4	Holalakere(1)	19.74	16.15	63	86	–3.59
	5	Hosadurga(1)	28.26	23.26	27	40	–5.00
	6	Molakalmur(1)	14.26	38.59	98	8	24.33
2.Davanagere	1	Davanagere(2)	31.18	19.77	19	60	–11.41
	2	Harihara(2)	21.48	24.04	53	34	2.57
	3	Channagiri(2)	16.03	23.64	88	37	7.61
	4	Honnalli(2)	11.46	–35.01	115	143	–46.47
	5	Harapanahally(2)	20.03	18.52	62	72	–1.51
	6	Jagalur(2)	19.48	17.94	66	74	–1.54
3.Kolar	1	Bagepally(3)	35.77	38.68	12	7	2.91
	2	Bangarpet(3)	10.18	5.07	120	128	–5.11
	3	Chikkaballpur(3)	15.09	14.09	95	97	–0.99
	4	Chintamani(3)	22.20	23.05	48	42	0.86
	5	Gauribidanoor(3)	23.14	–4.89	44	136	–28.04
	6	Gudibanda(3)	15.13	14.13	94	96	–1.00
	7	Kolar(3)	20.96	26.88	57	23	5.93
	8	Malur(3)	28.25	24.37	28	31	–3.89
	9	Mulbagil(3)	24.65	19.34	36	63	–5.32
	10	Sidlagatta(3)	10.67	38.74	119	6	28.07
	11	Srinivaspur(3)	24.88	27.91	34	17	3.04
4.Shimoga	1	Badravathi(4)	12.50	7.10	109	122	–5.40
	2	Hosanagar(4)	40.78	–52.73	6	145	–93.51
	3	Sagar(4)	6.43	11.50	131	108	5.07
	4	Shikaripur(4)	15.33	15.29	93	90	–0.04
	5	Shimoga(4)	20.95	27.73	58	19	6.78
	6	Sorab(4)	19.35	–11.62	67	139	–30.97
	7	Tirthahally(4)	7.01	11.59	128	106	4.58

Cont'd...

Cont'd...

5.Tumkur	1	C.N.Hally(5)	11.70	21.11	114	50	9.41
	2	Gubbi(5)	15.54	17.80	91	75	2.26
	3	Koratagere(5)	29.88	15.55	22	87	–14.33
	4	Kunigal(5)	22.19	23.44	49	38	1.24
	5	Madhugiri(5)	17.16	17.02	79	78	–0.15
	6	Pavagada(5)	23.79	–2.58	41	134	–26.37
	7	Sira(5)	17.15	33.33	80	10	16.18
	8	Tiptur(5)	15.49	32.11	92	12	16.62
	9	Tumkur(5)	39.59	27.74	8	18	–11.85
	10	Turuvekere(5)	24.71	8.77	35	117	–15.93
		II Belgaum division					
6.Belgaum	1	Athani(6)	85.83	21.76	1	47	–64.07
	2	Belgaum(6)	23.79	20.55	41	53	–3.24
	3	Chhikkodi(6)	16.96	14.93	81	92	–2.03
	4	Gokak(6)	17.86	10.31	75	113	–7.55
	5	Hukkeri(6)	19.26	6.53	68	125	–12.73
	6	Khanapur(6)	13.47	6.67	103	124	–6.80
	7	Parasgad(6)	20.32	13.15	60	99	–7.17
	8	Raibagh(6)	16.30	6.06	87	126	–10.25
	9	Ramadurga(6)	7.07	19.09	127	65	12.03
	10	Sampagon(6)	21.97	21.54	51	49	–0.43
7.Bijapur	1	Basavana b.wadi(7)	18.03	19.39	73	62	1.36
	2	Bijapur(7)	23.72	23.93	42	36	0.21
	3	Indi(7)	29.27	20.21	24	55	–9.07
	4	Muddebihal (7)	20.67	22.87	59	43	2.20
	5	Sindgi(7)	2.30	41.65	135	4	39.35
8.Bagalkote	1	Badami(8)	16.79	10.35	83	112	–6.43
	2	Bagalkot(8)	11.76	15.48	113	89	3.72
	3	Bilgi(8)	0.00	0.00	—	—	0.00
	4	Hungund(8)	–11.18	20.68	142	52	31.86
	5	Jamkhandi(8)	13.30	16.91	106	79	3.61
	6	Mudhol(8)	–25.95	26.77	145	24	52.72
9.Dharwad	1	Dharwad(9)	10.07	11.08	121	109	1.01
	2	Kalgatgi(9)	0.00	0.00	—	—	0.00
	3	Kundgol(9)	2.61	12.65	134	102	10.04
	4	Hubli(9)	0.00	0.00	—	—	0.00
	5	Navalgund(9)	23.07	6.75	45	123	–16.31

Cont'd...

Cont'd...

10.Gadag	1	Mundargi(10)	17.68	18.76	77	68	1.08
	2	Naragund(10)	21.42	8.04	54	119	–13.38
	3	Ron(10)	12.30	13.01	110	100	0.72
	4	Shirhatti(10)	11.46	11.80	115	104	0.34
	5	Gadag(10)	11.95	13.44	111	98	1.49
11. Haveri	1	Hangal(11)	18.26	16.41	72	83	–1.85
	2	Haveri(11)	19.71	18.99	64	66	–0.72
	3	Hirekerur(11)	0.00	0.00	—	—	0.00
	4	Byadgi(11)	12.83	19.83	107	59	7.00
	5	Ranibennur(11)	13.83	30.00	102	15	16.18
	6	Savanur(11)	15.76	16.38	90	85	0.62
	7	Shiggon(11)	24.35	55.64	37	2	31.28
12.Uttara Kannada	1	Ankola(12)	10.04	48.32	122	3	38.28
	2	Bhatkal(12)	18.47	25.30	71	28	6.84
	3	Haliyal(12)	–2.80	5.62	140	127	8.42
	4	Honnavar(12)	6.60	9.16	129	115	2.56
	5	Karwar(12)	22.44	18.89	47	67	–3.55
	6	Kumta(12)	10.68	24.11	118	33	13.43
	7	Mundgol(12)	0.00	0.00	—	—	0.00
	8	Siddapur(12)	0.00	0.00	—		0.00
	9	Sirsi(12)	23.55	22.10	43	45	–1.45
	10	Supa(12)	0.00	0.00	—	—	0.00
	11	Yellapur(12)	22.70	14.89	46	93	–7.80
		III Gulbarga division					
13.Bellary	1	Bellary(13)	17.85	22.53	76	44	4.68
	2	Hadagali(13)	26.66	20.08	33	57	–6.58
	3	H.B. hally(13)	0.00	0.00	—	—	0.00
	4	Hospet(13)	14.49	15.54	97	88	1.05
	5	Kudaligi(13)	–53.47	56.96	147	1	110.43
	6	Sandur(13)	–25.74	–33.76	145	142	–8.02
	7	Siruguppa(13)	24.03	24.58	39	30	0.55
14.Bidar	1	Aurad(14)	0.00	0.00	—	—	0.00
	2	Basavakalyna(14)	22.11	27.28	50	21	5.17
	3	Bhalki(14)	29.95	23.41	21	39	–6.53
	4	Bidar(14)	40.44	24.01	7	35	–16.43
	5	Homnabad(14)	11.92	28.33	112	16	16.41

Cont'd...

Cont'd...

15.Gulbarga	1	Afzalpur(15)	0.00	0.00	—	—	0.00
	2	Aland(15)	0.49	24.63	137	29	24.14
	3	Chincholli(15)	1.42	38.26	136	9	36.85
	4	Chitapur(15)	13.37	21.64	104	48	8.26
	5	Gulbarga(15)	28.82	27.74	26	18	–1.08
	6	Jevargi(15)	0.00	0.00	—	—	0.00
	7	Sedam(15)	52.43	17.10	2	77	–35.33
	8	Shahapur(15)	43.44	27.25	4	22	–16.18
	9	Shorapur(15)	34.07	11.00	14	110	–23.08
	10	Yadgir(15)	8.99	24.29	124	32	15.30
16.Raichur	1	Devadurga(16)	20.22	31.99	61	13	11.77
	2	Lingasugur(16)	37.73	16.40	10	84	–21.33
	3	Manvi(16)	23.99	25.34	40	27	1.36
	4	Raichur(16)	31.88	19.11	18	64	–12.77
	5	Sindanoor(16)	41.69	27.57	5	20	–14.12
	6	Gangavathi(16)	27.63	19.96	31	58	–7.67
17.Koppal	1	Koppal(17)	16.87	18.69	82	70	1.82
	2	Kustagi(17)	19.59	30.83	65	14	11.24
	3	Yelbarga(17)	0.00	0.00	—	—	0.00
		IV Mysore division					
18.Chickmagalur	1	Chickmagalur(18)	0.38	39.94	138	5	39.55
	2	Kadur(18)	17.59	15.00	78	91	–2.58
	3	Koppa(18)	5.24	1.78	132	131	–3.46
	4	Mudigere(18)	4.38	7.74	133	120	3.35
	5	N.R.Pura(18)	6.47	12.59	130	103	6.13
	6	Sringeri(18)	–3.04	2.42	141	130	5.46
	7	Tarikere(18)	7.33	–0.16	126	132	–7.49
19.Dakshin Kannada	1	Bantval(19)	29.57	18.73	23	69	–10.85
	2	Belthangadi(19)	0.00	0.00	—	—	0.00
	3	Mangalore(19)	21.86	26.72	52	25	4.87
	4	Puttur(19)	38.29	32.23	9	11	–6.07
	5	Sulya(19)	0.00	0.00	—	—	0.00
20.Udupi	1	Karkal(20)	14.23	–59.17	99	146	–73.39
	2	Kundapur(20)	8.54	–85.17	125	148	–93.71
	3	Udupi(20)	44.20	4.60	3	129	–39.60

Cont'd...

Cont'd...

21.Hassan	1	Alur(21)	15.80	19.11	89	64	3.31
	2	Arkalgud(21)	15.13	–39.82	94	144	–54.95
	4	Belur(21)	19.24	16.81	69	80	–2.42
	5	Channaraya(21)	21.11	20.16	56	56	–0.95
	6	Hassan(21)	32.50	14.66	16	95	–17.84
	7	Holenarsipur(21)	14.21	12.79	100	101	–1.41
	8	Sakaleshpur(21)	36.28	18.57	11	71	–17.71
22.Kodagu	1	Madikeri(22)	14.00	11.53	101	107	–2.48
	2	Somavarpet(22)	–1.29	–23.40	139	140	–22.11
	3	virajpet(22)	10.73	–6.81	117	138	–17.53
23. Mandya	1	Krishnarajpet(23)	28.88	20.29	25	54	–8.60
	2	Maddur(23)	21.31	16.61	55	81	–4.70
	3	Malavalli(23)	15.08	–3.50	96	135	–18.57
	4	Mandya(23)	16.61	8.32	84	118	–8.29
	5	Nagamangala(23)	18.54	–26.36	70	141	–44.90
	6	Pandavapura(23)	11.06	–5.14	116	137	–16.21
	7	Srirangapatna(23)	–11.32	7.69	143	121	19.00
24.Mysore	1	H.D.Kote(24)	31.89	–66.97	17	147	–98.86
	2	Hunsur(24)	20.22	20.84	61	51	0.62
	3	Krishnarajnag(24)	27.70	14.85	30	94	–12.85
	4	Mysore(24)	26.67	18.25	32	73	–8.42
	5	Nanjangud(24)	17.98	11.68	74	105	–6.30
	6	Piriyapatna(24)	16.40	19.54	86	61	3.14
	7	T.narasipur(24)	13.35	16.42	105	82	3.07
25.Chamaraj-nagar	1	Chamarajnagar(25)	9.12	26.55	123	26	17.43
	2	Gundlupet(25)	16.58	9.13	85	116	–7.45
	3	Kollegal(25)	24.12	9.55	38	114	–14.57
	4	Yelndur(25)	12.61	!0.56	108	111	–2.04
Karnataka			22.85	22.38	—	—	–0.47

Source: 1. Census of India 1981 series–9 Karnataka, 2.Census of India 1991 Karnataka series 11, 3. Census C.D.s Registrar General of India 2001.

Note: For both the decades the urban population data are not available for 14 taluks.
3 taluks in the decade 1981-1991 fall under same rank (Urban population)
2 taluks in the decade 1991-2001 fall under same rank.

Annexure 4

Taluks of Very High (VH) Growth Rate in the Decade 1981–1991

District	*S.No.*	*Taluk*
Bagalkot	1	Badami
	2	Bilgi
	3	Jhamkhandi
	4	Mudhol
Bellary	5	Bellary
	6	Hadagali
	7	H.B. Hally
	8	Hospet
	9	Kudligi
	10	Sandur
	11	Siruguppa
Belgaum	12	Athani
	13	Belgaum
	14	Gokak
	15	Parasgad
	16	Raybag
	17	Ramdurga
	18	Sampagan
Bidar	19	Aurad
	20	Basavakalyana
	21	Bhalki
	22	Bidar
	23	Homnabad
Bijapur	24	Bijapur
	25	Indi
	26	Muddebihal
	27	Sindgi
Chitradurga	28	Challakere
	29	Chitradurga
	30	Molakalmur
Dharwad	31	Dharwad
	32	Kalghatgi

Cont'd...

Cont'd...

Dakshin Kannada	33	Belthangadi
	34	Puttur
	35	Sulya
Davanagere	36	Davanagere
	37	Harihara
	38	Harapanahally
	39	Jagalure
Gadag	40	Naragund
Gulbarga	41	Afzalpur
	42	Aland
	43	Chincholli
	44	Chitapur
	45	Gulbarga
	46	Jevargi
	47	Sedam
	48	Shahapur
	49	Shorapur
	50	Yadgir
Hassan	51	Arkalgud
	52	Hassan
	53	Holenarasipur
Haveri	54	Hangal
	55	Haveri
	56	Hirekerur
	57	Byadgi
	58	Ranibennur
	59	Savanur
	60	Shiggon
Kolar	61	Chikkaballapur
	62	Chintamani
	63	Malur
	64	Mulbagil
Koppal	65	Koppal
	66	Kustagi
	67	Yelbarga

Cont'd...

Cont'd...

Mandya	68	K.R. Pet
Mysore	69	H.D. Kote
	70	Hunsur
	71	K.R. Nagar
	72	Mysore
	73	Nanjangud
	74	Piriyapatna
Raichur	75	Devadurga
	76	Lingasugur
	77	Manvi
	78	Raichur
	79	Sindanur
	80	Gangavathi
Shimoga	81	Shikaripura
	82	Shimoga
Tumkur	83	Tumkur
	84	Sira
Uttar Kannada	85	Bhatkal
	86	Mundgod

Annexure 5

Demoted Taluks from VH Level (1981–1991) Growth to H and M Levels

District	S.No.	Taluk
Bagalkot	1	Badami
Bellary	2	Hadagali
Belgaum	3	Parasgad
	4	Ramdurga
	5	Sampagan
Bidar	6	Aurad
	7	Bhalki
Bijapur	8	Indi
	9	Muddebihal
	10	Sindgi
Chitradurga	11	Chitradurga
Dharwad	12	Dharwad
	13	Kalghatgi
Dakshin Kannada	14	Belthangadi
	15	Puttur
	16	Sulya
Davanagere	17	Davanagere
	18	Harihara
	19	Harapanahally
	20	Jagalure
Gadag	21	Naragund *
Gulbarga	22	Aland
Hassan	23	Arkalgud *
	24	Holenarasipur *
	25	Hassan
Haveri	26	Hangal
	27	Haveri
	28	Hirekerur *

Cont'd...

Cont'd...

	29	Byadgi
	30	Ranibennur
	31	Savanur
	32	Shiggon
Kolar	33	Chikkaballapur
	34	Chintamani
	35	Mulbagil
Mandya	36	K.R. Pet
Mysore	37	H.D. Kote
	38	Hunsur
	39	K.R. Nagar
Shimoga	40	Shikaripura
Uttar Kannada	41	Bhatkal

Note: * Shows taluk depromoted to M Level.

Annexure 6

Taluks Continued as VH Level in Both the Decades 1981–1991 and 1991–2001

District	S.No	Taluk
Chitradurga	1	Challakere
	2	Molakalmur
Kolar	3	Kolar*
	4	Malur
Shimoga	5	Shimoga
Tumkur	6	Tumkur
	7	Sira
Belgaum	8	Athani
	9	Belgaum
	10	Gokak
	11	Raybag
Bijapur	12	Bijapur
	13	B.B. Vadi
Bagalkot	14	Bagalkot*
	15	Bilgi
	16	Jamkhandi
	17	Mudhol
Uttar Kannada	18	Mundgol
Bellary	19	Bellary
	20	Hospet
	21	Kudligi
	22	Sandur
	23	Siruguppa
	24	H.B. Hally
Bidar	25	Basavakalyana
	26	Bidar
	27	Homnabad

Cont'd...

Cont'd...

Gulbarga	28	Afzalpur
	29	Chincholli
	30	Chitapur
	31	Gulbarga
	32	Jevargi
	33	Shahapur
	34	Shorapur
	35	Yadgir
	36	Sedam
Raichur	37	Devadurga
	38	Lingasugur
	39	Manvi
	40	Raichur
	41	Sindanur
	42	Gangavathi
Koppal	43	Koppal
	44	Kustagi
	45	Yelbarga
Dakshin Kannada	46	Mangalore*
Mysore	47	Mysore
	48	Piriyapatna

Note: *Taluk promoted to VH from H Level.

Annexure 7
Taluks of VH Level Growth Rate in Rural Population in the Decade 1981–1991

District	*Taluk*
Chitradurga	1. Challakere
	2. Molakalmur
Davanagere	3. Harihara
	4. Harapanahally
	5. Jagalur
Kolar	6. Chikkaballapur
	7. Malur
	8. Sidlagatta
Shimoga	9. Shikaripur
	10. Shimoga
Tumkur	11. Sira
Belgaum	12. Athani
	13. Gokak
	14. Parasgad
	15. Raibagh
	16. Ramdurga
	17. Sampagon
Bijapur	18. Bijapur
	19. Indi
	20. Sindgi
Bagalkot	21. Bilgi
	22. Hungund
	23. Jamkhandi
	24. Mudhol
	25. Badami
Dharwad	26. Dharwad
	27. Kalgatgi

Cont'd...

Cont'd...

Gadag	28. Naragund
Haveri	29. Hangal
	30. Haveri
	31. Hirekerur
	32. Byadgi
	33. Ranibennur
	34. Savanur
	35. Shiggon
Uttar Kannada	36. Bhatkal
	37. Mundgod
	38. Siddapur
Bellary	39. Bellary
	40. Hadagali
	41. H.B. Hally
Bidar	42. Hospet
	43. Kudligi
	44. Sandur
	45. Siruguppa
	50. Homnabad
Gulbarga	51. Afzalpur
	52. Aland
	53. Chicholli
	54. Chitapur
	55. Jevargi
	56. Shahapur
	57. Shorapur
	58. Yadgir
Raichur	59. Devadurga
	60. Lingasugur
	61. Manvi

Cont'd...

Cont'd...

	62. Raichur
	63. Sindanur
	64. Gangavathi
Koppal	65. Koppal
	66. Kustagi
	67. Yelabarga
Dakshin Kannada	68. Belthangadi
	69. Sulya
Hassan	70. Arkalgud
	71. Holenarasipur
Mandya	72. Pandavapur
Mysore	73. H.D. Kote
	74. Hunsur
	75. Mysore
	76. Nanjangud
	77. Piriyapatna

Annexure 8

Taluks of VH Level Growth Rate in Rural Population in the Decade 1991–2001

District	***Taluk***
Chitradurga	1. Challakere
	2. Molakalmur
Tumkur	3. Pavagada
Belgaum	4. Athani
	5. Gokak
	6. Raibagh
Bagalkot	7. Bagalkot
	8. Jamkhandi
	9. Mudhol
Bellary	10. Bellary
	11. Hospet
	12. Siruguppa
	13. Basavakalyna
Gulbarga	14. Shahapur
	15. Shorapur
	16. Sedam
Raichur	17. Devadurga
	18. Lingasugur
	19. Manvi
	20. Raichur
	21. Sindanur
	22. Gangavathi
Koppal	23. Koppal
	24. Kustagi
Dakshin Kannada	25. Mangalore
Udupi	26. Kundapur
Kodagu	27. Somavarpet
Mysore	28. H.D. Kote
	29. Mysore
	30. Piriyapatna

Annexure 9

Demoted Taluks from VH Level Growth Rate in Rural Population to H,M, and Low Levels in the Decade 1991–2001

District	*Taluk*	*Level*
Davanagere	1. Harihara	Low
	2. Harapanahally	High
	3. Jagalur	High
Kolar	4. Chikkaballapur	High
	5. Malur	High
	6. Sidlagatta	Low
Shimoga	7. Shikaripur	High
	8. Shimoga	Low
Tumkur	9. Sira	High
Belgaum	10. Parasgad	High
	11. Ramdurga	Medium
	12. Sampagon	High
Bijapur	13. Bijapur	High
	14. Indi	High
	15. Sindgi	High
Bagalkot	16. Bilgi	Low
	17. Hungund	High
	18. Badami	High
Dharwad	19. Dharwad	High
	20. Kalghatgi	Low
Gadag	21. Naragund	Low
Haveri	22. Haveri	High
	23. Hangal	High
	24. Hirekerur	Low
	25. Byadgi	High
	26. Ranibennur	Low
	27. Savanur	High
	28. Shiggon	Negative
Uttar Kannada	29. Bhatkal	Medium
	30. Mundgod	Negative

Cont'd...

Cont'd...

	31. Siddapur	Negative
Bellary	32. Hadagali	High
	33. Kudligi	High
	34. Sandur	Negative
Bidar	35. Aurad	High
	36. Bidar	High
	37. Homnabad	High
Gulbarga	38. Afzalpur	Medium
	39. Aland	High
	40. Chicholli	High
	41. Chitapur	High
	42. Jevargi	High
Gulbarga	43. Yadgir	High
Koppal	44. Yelabarga	High
Dakshin Kannada	45. Belthangadi	High
	46. Sulya	Negative
Hassan	47. Arkalgud	High
	48. Holenarasipur	Medium
Mandya	49. Pandavapura	High
Mysore	50. Hunsur	High
	51. Nanjangud	Medium

Annexure 10

Taluks of VH Level Growth Rate of Rural Population in both the Decade

District	*Taluk*
Chitradurga	1. Challakere
	2. Molakalmur
Belgaum	3. Athani
	4. Gokak
	5. Raibagh
Bagalkot	6. Jamkhandi
	7. Mudhol
Bellary	8. Bellary
	9. H.B. Hally
	10. Hospet
	11. Siruguppa
Bidar	12. Basavakalyana
Gulbarga	13. Shahapur
	14. Shorapur
Raichur	15. Devadurga
	16. Lingasugur
	17. Manvi
	18. Raichur
	19. Sindanur
	20. Gangavathi
Koppal	21. Koppal
	22. Kustagi
Mysore	23. H.D. Kote
	24. Mysore
	25. Piriyapatna

Annexure 11

Promoted Taluks in Growth of Urban Population from High to Very High Level in Decade1991–2001 from Previous Decade

District	*Taluk*
Tumkur	Pavagada
Bagalkot	Bagalkot
Gulbarga	Sedam
Dakshin Kannada	Mangalore
Udupi	Kundapur
Kodagu	Somavarpet

Annexure 12

Taluks of VH Level Growth Rate in Urban Population in the Decade 1981–1991

District	*Taluk*
Chitradurga	1. Challakere
	2. Chitradurga
	3. Hiriyur
	4. Holalkere
	5. Hosadurga
Davanagere	6. Davanagere
	7. Harihara
	8. Channagiri
	9. Harapanahally
	10. Jagalur
Kolar	11. Bagepally
	12. Chintamani
	13. Kolar
	14. Malur
	15. Mulbagil
	16. Srinivaspura

Cont'd...

Cont'd...

	17. Chikkaballapur
	18. Gouribidanur
	19. Gudibanda
Shimoga	20. Hosanagar
	21. Shikaripur
	22. Shimoga
	23. Sorab
Tumkur	24. Gubbi
	25. Koratagere
	26. Kunigal
	27. Madhugiri
	28. Pavagada
	29. Sira
	30. Tiptur
	31. Tumkur
	32. Turuvekere
Belgaum	33. Athani
	34. Belgaum
	35. Chikkodi
	36. Gokak
	37. Hukkeri
	38. Parasgad
	39. Raibagh
	40. Sampagon
Bijapur	41. B.B. Vadi
	42. Bijapur
	43. Indi
	44. Muddebihal
Bagalkot	45. Badami
Dharwad	46. Navalgund

Cont'd...

Cont'd...

Gadag	47. Mundargi
	48. Naragund
Haveri	49. Hangal
	50. Haveri
	51. Savanur
	52. Shiggon
Uttar Kannada	53. Bhatkal
	54. Karwar
	55. Sirsi
	56. Yellapur
Bellary	57. Bellary
	58. Hadagali
	59. Siruguppa
Bidar	60. Basavakalyna
	61. Bhalki
	62. Bidar
Gulbarga	63. Gulbarga
	64. Sedam
	65. Shahapur
	66. Shorapur
Raichur	67. Devadurga
	68. Lingasugur
	69. Manvi
	70. Raichur
	71. Sindanur
	72. Gangavathi
Koppal	73. Koppal
	74. Kustagi
Chickmagalur	75. Chickmagalur
Dakshin Kannada	76. Bantval

Cont'd...

Cont'd...

	77. Mangalore
	78. Puttur
Udupi	79. Udupi
Hassan	80. Alur
	81. Arkalgud
	82. Arasikere
	83. Channarayapatna
	84. Hassan
	85. Sakaleshwar
	86. Belur
Mandya	87. K.R. Pet
	88. Maddur
	89. Malavalli
	90. Mandya
	91. Nagamangala
Mysore	92. H.D. Kote
	93. Hunsur
	94. Krishnaraj Nagar
	95. Mysore
	96. Nanjangud
	97. Piriyapatna
Chamarajnagar	98. Gundlupet
	99. Kollegal

Annexure 13

Demoted Taluks in Growth of Urban Population from VH Level to H, M, and Low Levels in Decade 1991–2001 from Previous Decade

District	*Taluk*
Kolar	1. Chikkaballapur
	2. Gouribidanur
	3. Gudibanda
Shimoga	4. Hosanagar
	5. Sorab
Tumkur	6. Pavagada
	7. Turuvekere
Belgaum	8. Chikkodi
	9. Hukkeri
	10. Parasgad
	11. Raibagh
	12. Gokak
Bagalkot	13. Badami
Dharwad	14. Navalgund
Naragund	15. Naragund
Uttar Kannada	16. Yellapur
Gulbarga	17. Shorapur
Udupi	18. Udupi
Hassan	19. Arkalgud
	20. Hassan
Mandya	21. Mandya
	22. Nagamangala
Mysore	23. H.D. Kote
	24. K.R. Nagar
	25. Nanjangud
Chamarajnagar	26. Gundlupet
	27. Kollegal

Annexure 14

Taluks Remained in VH Level Growth Rate in Urban Population in both the Decades

District	*Taluk*
Chitradurga	1. Challakere
	2. Chitrdurga
	3. Hiriyur
	4. Holalkere
	5. Hosadurga
Davanagere	6. Davanagere
	7. Harihara
	8. Channagiri
	9. Harapanahally
	10. Jagalur
Kolar	11. Bagepalli
	12. Chintamani
	13. Kolar
	14. Malur
	15. Mulbagil
	16. Srinivasapur
Shimoga	17. Shikaripura
	18. Shimoga
Tumkur	19. Gubbi
	20. Koratagere
	21. Kunigal
	22. Madhugiri
	23. Sira
	24. Tiptur
	25. Tumkur
Belgaum	26. Athani
	27. Belgaum
	28. Sampagon
Bijapur	29. B.B. Vadi
	30. Bijapur

Cont'd...

Cont'd...

	31. Indi
	32. Muddebihal
Gadag	33. Mundargi
Haveri	34. Hangal
	35. Haveri
	36. Savanur
	37. Shiggon
Uttar Kannada	38. Bhatkal
	39. Karwar
	40. Sirsi
Bellary	41. Bellary
	42. Hadagali
	43. Siruguppa
Bidar	44. Basavakalyna
	45. Bhalki
	46. Bidar
Gulbarga	47. Gulbarga
	48. Sedam
	49. Shahapur
	50. Shorapur
Raichur	51. Devadurga
	52. Lingasugur
	53. Manvi
	54. Raichur
	55. Sindanur
	56. Gangavathi
Koppal	57. Koppal
	58. Kustagi
Chickmagalur	59. Kadur
Dakshin Kannada	60. Bantval
	61. Mangalore
	62. Puttur
Hassan	63. Alur

Cont'd...

Cont'd...

	64. Arasikere
	65. Channarayapatna
	66. Belur
	67. Sakaleshwar
Mandya	68. K.R. Pet
	69. Maddur
Mysore	70. Hunsur
	71. Mysore
	72. Piriyapatna

Annexure 15

Promoted Taluks in Growth of Urban Population from Lower to Higher (VH) Level in Decade 1991–2001 from Previous Decade

District	***Taluk***
Chitradurga	1. Molakalmur(H)
Kolar	2. Sidlagatta(H)
Tumkur	3. C.N. Hally(H)
Belgaum	4. Ramdurga(M)
Bijapur	5. Sindgi(L)
Bagalkot	6. Bagalkot(H)
	7. Jhamkhandi(H)
Haveri	8. Byadgi(H)
	9. Ranibennur(H)
Uttar Kannada	10. Ankola(H)
	11. Kumta(H)
Bellary	12. Hospet(H)
Bidar	13. Humnabad(H)
	14. Aland(L)
	15. Chincholli(L)
	16. Chitapur(H)
	17. Yadgir(M)
Chickmagalur	18. Chickmagalur(L)
Mysore	19. T.Narasipur(H)
Chamarajnagar	20.Chamarajnagar(M)

Annexure 16

Scoring Order for Selected Health Care Indicators for Children's Health Care Infrastructure Index in Karnataka

A. Health Care Infrastructure

S.No.	*District*	*No. of wards*	*No. of beds*	*No. of working doctors*	*NICU facility*	*Well-baby clinic*	*Ultra sound*
1	Bagalkot	1	1	0	0	0	0
2	Bellary	2	2	1	1	0	1
3	Belgaum	1	2	2	1	0	1
4	Bidar	3	1	1	0	0	1
5	Bijapur	1	1	0	0	0	1
6	Chamarajnagar	1	1	1	0	0	1
7	Chickmagalur	1	1	1	1	0	1
8	Chitradurga	1	2	1	1	0	1
9	Davanagere	2	3	1	1	1	1
10	Dharwad	1	2	1	1	0	1
11	Dakshin Kannada	2	2	1	1	1	1
12	Gadag	1	1	1	0	0	1
13	Gulbarga	2	3	2	1	0	1
14	Haveri	1	1	0	0	0	1
15	Hassn	1	1	1	1	0	1
16	Kolar	3	1	1	0	1	1
17	Koppal	1	1	0	0	0	1
18	Kodagu	1	1	1	1	0	1
19	Mandya	2	1	1	1	0	0
20	Mysore	2	2	1	1	1	1
21	Raichur	2	1	1	1	0	1
22	Shimoga	1	1	1	1	0	1
23	Tumkur	1	1	1	1	0	1
24	Udupi	1	2	1	0	0	1
25	Uttar Kannada	1	1	1	1	0	1

B. Health Care Facilities

S.No.	District	Laser	Fibre optic dndo-scopy	Micro-scope	Total scoring	Proportion of child popula-ti on	Rank
1	Bagalkot	1	0	1	4	16	2
2	Bellary	1	1	1	10	15.7	4
3	Belgaum	0	0	1	9	14.8	5
4	Bidar	0	0	1	7	16	2
5	Bijapur	0	0	1	4	15.8	3
6	Chamarajnagar	1	1	0	6	12	14
7	Chickmagalur	1	0	0	6	12.2	13
8	Chitradurga	1	0	0	7	13	10
9	Davanagere	1	1	1	12	13.4	9
10	Dharwad	1	0	0	7	13.6	8
11	Dakshin Kanada	1	1	1	11	12	14
12	Gadag	1	0	0	5	14	7
13	Gulbarga	0	0	1	10	17	1
14	Haveri	1	0	0	4	14.2	6
15	Hassn	1	1	0	7	11.6	15
16	Kolar	0	0	1	8	13.2	10
17	Koppal	1	0	0	4	17	1
18	Kodagu	1	1	0	7	12.6	12
19	Mandya	0	0	0	5	11.6	15
20	Mysore	1	1	1	11	12.2	13
21	Raichur	0	0	1	7	17	1
22	Shimoga	1	1	0	7	12.6	12
23	Tumkur	0	1	1	7	12	14
24	Udupi	1	1	0	7	10.3	16
25	Uttar Kannada	1	1	1	8	12.8	11

Note: Derived from Tables 3.1, 3.2 and 3.4

Scoring order

—Each children ward scoring 1, score 1 for 10–30 beds, 31–60, scoring is 2 and 61–90 scoring is 3, If NICU facility exiting scoring order is 1, if no existing, 0

If well-baby clinic facility exiting scoring order is 1, if no, 0

If modern equipments provided score is 1, if no, 0

Annexure 17
Children's Health Care Infrastructure Index by Districts in Karnataka

Relatively Good (Scoring 8 to 12)	1. Davanagere
	2. Dakshin Kannada
	3. Mysore
	4. Bellary
	5. Gulbarga
	6. Belgaum
	7. Kolar
	8. Uttar Kannada
Relatively Moderate (Scoring 5 to 7)	9. Bidar
	10. Chitradurga
	11. Dharwad
	12. Hassan
	13. Kodagu
	14. Raichur
	15. Shimoga
	16. Udupi
	17. Chamarajnagar
	18. Chickmagalur
	19. Gadag
	20. Mandya
Relatively Low (Scoring below 4)	21. Bagalkot
	22. Bijapur
	23. Haveri
	24. Koppal

Note: Computed from Table 7.1.

Annexure 18

Rank Order of Districts in Proportion of Child Population in Karnataka

High Proportion(First order of ranks from 1–5)	1. Gulbarga
	2. Koppal
	3. Raichur
	4. Bagalkot
	5. Bidar
	6. Bijapur
	7. Bellary
	8. Belgaum
Medium Proportion(Second order of ranks from 6–10)	9. Haveri
	10. Gadag
	11. Dharwad
	12. Davanagere
	13. Chitradurga
	14. Kolar
Low Proportion(Third order of ranks from 11–15)	15. Uttar Kannada
	16. Shimoga
	17. Kodagu
	18. Chickmagalur
	19. Mysore
	20. Chamarajnagar
	21. Dakshin Kannada
	22. Hassan
	23. Mandya
	24. Udupi

Source Derived from Annexure 16.

References

Betteile, Andre (2000). *Essays on Ideologies and Institutions*, Oxford University Press, New Delhi.

Bhagat, R.B. and Aparajita Chattopadhya (2004). "Characteristics and Correlates of Tribal Fertility: A Comparative Study of Selected Tribes", *Demography India*, Vol. 33, No. 2.

Bhattacharjee, P.J. (1978). *Population in India*, Vikas, New Delhi.

Bose, Ashish et al. (1967). *Patterns of Population Change in India 1951–1961*, Allied Publishers, Bombay.

Carneiro, Robert L., ed. 1967. *The Evolution of Society: Selected from Herbert Spencer's Principles of Sociology*. Chicago: University of Chicago Press.

Castro, Josue De (1952). *The Geography of Hunger*, Hermitage House, New York.

Chaudhury, Debadutta and S.N. Tripathy (2005). *Girl Child and Human Rights*. Anmol Publications, New Delhi.

Clark, Colin (1970). *Population Growth and Land Use*, MacMillan and Co. Ltd., London.

Davis, Adelle (1959). *Let's Have Healthy Children*, Unwin Books, London.

De Souza, Alfred et al. (1979). *Children in India*. Manohar Publications, New Delhi.

Goswami, Homeswar (1985). *Population Trends in the Brahmaputra Valley*, Delhi, Mittal Publications.

Government of India (1986). Statistical Abstract, Central Statistical Organisation, Department of Statistics, New Delhi.

—— (1991 and 2001). Statistical Abstract–India Central Statistical Organization, New Delhi.

—— (2000). National Population Policy 2000. Ministry of Health and Family Welfare, New Delhi.

—— (2001). Reproductive Child Health Report Phase I and II (1992–1993 and 1998–1999). Ministry of Health and Family Welfare, New Delhi.

Government of Karnataka (2001). Karnataka at a Glance, Directorate of Economics and Statistics, Bangalore, Government of Karnataka.

—— (2002). Districtwise District at a Glance, Directorate of Economics and Statistics, Bangalore.

—— (2002). Final Report of the High Power Committee for Redressal of Regional Imbalances, Bangalore: Government of Karnataka.

—— (2002). Karnataka Socio-Economic Indicators, Directorate of Economics and Statistics, Bangalore.

Gulimoto and Rajan Irudaya (2001). Spatial Patterns of Fertility Transition in Indian Districts. *Population and Development Review*, XXXVII (7): 665-72.

Husain and Ishrat (1972). *Population Analysis and Studies*, Bombay, Somaiya Publications.

International Institute for Population Sciences (IIPS), 1995. National Family Health Survey (NFHS–2), Mumbai, IIPS

Jhingan, M.L., B.K. Bhatt and J.N. Desai (2003) *Demography*, Vrinda Publications (Pvt.) Ltd. New Delhi.

Kapur, R.S. and K.A. George (eds) (1965). Population Growth in Kerala, Bureau of Economics and Statistics, Trivandrum, Government of Kerala.

Kumar, Ashok et al. (1990). *Developing Women and Children in India*. Commonwealth Publishers, New Delhi.

Kurup, R.S. and K.A. George (eds.) (1964). Population Growth in Kerala, Bureau of Economics and Statistics, Trivandrum, Government of Kerala.

Kuznets, Simon (1974). Population Redistribution and Economic Growth in United States 1870-1950, American Philosophical Society, Philadelphia.

Lakshmana, C.M. (1998) Population Change and Socio-economic Development of Tumkur District, Ph.D thesis submitted to the Bangalore University, Bangalore.

—— (2005), Spatial Dimensions of Literacy and Index of Development in Karnataka, Working Paper No. 163, Institute for Social and Economic Change, Bangalore.

—— (2006). Population Change in Karnataka, Project Report submitted to ISEC. Bangalore.

Lee, Luke L. and Arthur Larsen (1971). *Population and Law*, Rule of Law Press, Durham.

Maharatna, Arup (2005). *Demographic Perspective on India's Tribes*, Oxford University Press, New Delhi.

Malthus, Thomas Robert (1965). *First Essay on Population*, Sentry Press, New York.

Mathur, Harimohan (eds) (1995). *Family Welfare Programs in India*, New Delhi: Vikas Publishing House.

Mehta, B.C. (1970) *Regional Population Growth*, Moonlight Printers, Jaipur.

Mukherjee, Ramakrishna (1976). *Family and Planning in India*, Orient Longman Ltd. Publications, Bombay.

Muthurayappa, R. (2000). *Tribal Fertility, Mortality and Health Care Practices*, Mittal Publications, New Delhi.

Nanjundappa, D.M. (2002). Final Report of the High Power Committee for Redressal of Regional Imbalances in Karnataka, Bangalore, Government of Karnataka.

Pathak, Lalit P.(1998) *Population Studies*, Rawat Publications, New Delhi.

Patil, R.N. (1978) *Population, Family and Culture*, Ashish Publishing House, New Delhi.

Population Census Abstract.1991 and 2001.Census of India. New Delhi.

Population Research Centre, ISEC, Bangalore: RCH Project Report Rapid Household Survey, Karnataka 1992 and 1998.

Raha, Manis Kumar et al. (1989). *Tribal India*, Gyan Publishing House, New Delhi.

Ramachanrudu (1989). *Determinants of Population Growth in India*, Inter–India Publications, New Delhi.

Rayappa, P.H., T.V. Sekher and M. Ramakrishna Reddy (1998). Population Policy for Karnataka: A Suggested Framework, ISEC Working Paper No. 75, Bangalore, Institute for Social and Economic Change.

Registrar General and Census Commissioner, India 1991. Census of India, Series 1 Part–VIII–A & B (viii).

Registrar General: Population Census Abstract for the Year 1981, 1991 and 2001, New Delhi, Government of India.

Registrar General: Social and Cultural Tables for the Year 1981, 1991 and 2001. Census of India, New Delhi.

Sekher, T.V. (2006). Vulnerable Daughters in a Modernizing Society: From Son Preference to Daughter Discrimination in Rural India, Lund Working Paper Series, Lund University. Publishers, New Delhi.

Sekher, T.V. et al. (2001) "Fertility Transition in Karnataka: Levels Trends and Implications". *Economic and Political Weekly*, Vol XXXVI, No. 51.

Sekher, T.V., K.N.M. Raju and M.N. Sivakumar (2001). Fertility Transition in South India, Karnataka. In Government of Karnataka, Functional Review Reports, Bangalore: KARC.

Sekher, T.V. and K.N.M. Raju (2000), "Fertility Transition in Karnataka". Monograph No. 5, Institute for Social and Economic Change, Bangalore.

Singh, Ram Dayal (1985). *Population Structure of Indian Cities*, Inter-India Publications, New Delhi.

Sinha, Amarjeet (2005). *India*, Rupa and Company, New Delhi.

Vyas, Anju and Madhu Mudgal (1992). *The Girl Child in India*. Indian Bibliographies Bureau, New Delhi.

William (1967). *Famine 1975*, Little Brown and Company, Boston.

William, P O' Hare (2009). Comparing Child Poverty in America. Population Reference Bureau, New York.

Zelinsky, Wilbur (1966). *Prologue to Population Geography*, Printice-Hall of India Pvt Ltd., New Delhi.

Index